T0279865

How to Grow Through What You Go Through

Jodie Cariss and Chance Marshall

Vermilion

LONDON

1

Vermilion, an imprint of Ebury Publishing,
20 Vauxhall Bridge Road,
London SW1V 2SA

Vermilion is part of the Penguin Random House group of companies
whose addresses can be found at global.penguinrandomhouse.com

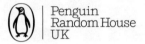

First published by Vermilion in 2022

www.penguin.co.uk

A CIP catalogue record for this book is available from the British Library

ISBN 9781785043680

Printed and bound in Great Britain by Clays Ltd, Elcograf S.p.A.

The authorised representative in the EEA is Penguin Random House Ireland,
Morrison Chambers, 32 Nassau Street, Dublin D02 YH68

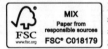

Penguin Random House is committed to a
sustainable future for our business, our readers
and our planet. This book is made from Forest
Stewardship Council® certified paper.

Contents

Introduction

We begin here with what we imagine is a shared curiosity: you curious enough about this book (and we hope yourself!) to pick it up, and us curious about you and why you might have found yourself here; not unlike a first therapy session, where we meet equally unknown to each other, where strangers arrive in the space with a hope of something. Sometimes the reason for arriving in therapy feels clear, sometimes not; sometimes people say they don't really know how they found us or they just had a feeling it was something they needed to do. Sometimes our clients come armed with a diagnosis they are terrified by or persistent symptoms they can't shift. They may be experiencing a life phase they can't get a handle on or an event they can't process. Or it could simply be that they want more energy, more boundaries, to make a good life better, more joy, more hope, more choice . . . the list is endless. But we always arrive ready to explore the very first question, as we are right now:

So what brings you here today?
What is it that you are hoping for as you
begin these pages?

Maybe life's feeling like a struggle. Perhaps nothing feels simple or easy any more. Maybe you are not exactly uncomfortable, but feel that you are not living all the way into the corners of yourself. Are you feeling lacklustre about work, parenting or your relationships? You might have worries – small or big – about your own mental health. Perhaps the motivation, meaning and purpose to life don't feel as obvious as they once did. Have you hit a significant milestone in your life and feel completely bewildered as to how or why you are here? You might be feeling anxious, upset, angry, frustrated, disillusioned, bored, griev-ing or overwhelmed by daily tasks. Or maybe life feels pretty good most of the time, but you have a sense that there is more potential to be actualised, good relationships to be made great, effective coping strategies to be diversified or good self-care to be made better. Perhaps you already understand the positive effects of working on your mental health and want a bit more guidance, a bit more of a push.

Whatever the reason, somewhere there is an interest in deepening your self-awareness and arming yourself with tools you might need at some point in time to help you stabilise. Somewhere, deep down, is an awareness that mental mainte-nance practices might enhance life for you.

It's a fact that life throws us many curveballs – unpreventable and unpredictable things happen all the time; some big, some small and everything in between. But often, much of what we feel is out of our control – as seemingly happening *to* us – is, in fact, the reality of what we create ourselves. We hope this book will give you some of the tools and a little of the courage it might take for you to create some positive changes in your life, to overcome that apathy we can so often feel about the place our life is in and to weather the storms that can sometimes hit us. With deep compassion, but with obvious challenge, we'll be inviting you to reflect on what has gone before and be more conscious of what is ahead, while also taking stock of what is happening right here, right now, as you read these words.

We can't 'grow through what we go through' if we don't have our eyes open to it all. We can't open our eyes to it all if we don't have the support and encouragement we need to really see what needs to be seen: the good, the less good and the damn near-impossible. Your better mental health is ultimately in your own hands – the power to challenge and encourage yourself to grow is with you at the core – but the journey can and should be shared. You need others, both for challenge and support. This book is a little of that. Like a good therapist who champions your wins and gives you a kick up the arse when you need it, think of us as walking with you, little voices on your shoulder when it feels hardest. Clients often say they hear the voices of their therapists when they feel most lost; sometimes that's annoying, sometimes it brings comfort. Reach out for this book when you need something to steady yourself or when you know you need a kick in the right direction.

About Us

Since our launch in 2017, Self Space – whose mission is to provide easy access to straightforward therapy, to both companies and individuals – has welcomed thousands of people through its doors and digital portals. Everyone who comes to us is different, all of the stories shared within our walls totally unique, but every teller is connected by their humanness and their desire to make more sense of themselves, their lives and the world around them. People might arrive tentative, nervous perhaps, afraid to reflect on their pasts, anxious, depressed, grieving, alone, yet eager to move forward, even excited about what might come. We welcome them all. But we never underestimate the abstractness of therapy and what we challenge our clients to do – to arrive in a space with a total stranger and bare their soul. To share truths they may not even have fully exposed themselves to. To sit in sometimes awkward silence, to allow themselves to be listened to, and be seen laughing, crying, confused and held for 50 minutes. A space where time can feel endless, or never enough, the gaze overwhelming. Yet our clients return, week after week, crossing thresholds, some big, some small, telling jokes, revealing memories, sharing photos, objects, wounds and more. All of them prepared to roll up their sleeves and do the work. How greatly we benefit from that courage. What an absolute honour it is to be surrounded by these people and immersed in their unfolding stories and call that our work. Because of that courage, we have the privilege to share a little of our learning from those emotional frontiers here in this book.

    None of us is exempt from the grind involved in maintaining our better mental health, yet so many of us place such unrealistically high expectations on ourselves. We hear clients say it all the time: 'I don't understand why I can't sort this out; I'm embarrassed to be here.' We imagine that, when we do hit choppy waters, which we all will in the course of our lives, we'll just automatically be able to swim, to sort it all out for ourselves. When you find you can't, or don't have the strength, stamina or internal resources to stay afloat, you feel let down by yourself. You might feel less than, confused, stressed, upset, helpless and hopeless, asking yourself, 'what is wrong with me?' People have a very unhelpful pre-programmed idea that we should be able to navigate life's challenges smoothly, without preparation, training or putting the work in. Yet you would not arrive at a marathon having never run before and expect to finish in good shape. So why expect the same of your mental health?

Almost everything we do is better when we apply ourselves, when we flex our muscles and build strength, when we prepare and ready ourselves – it gives us power and confidence in our resources. Preparation doesn't make you immune to poor mental health – hitting you at times like water in your face, big waves and changing tides – but confronting the difficult stuff on a day-to-day basis helps you to build stamina and mastery in understanding, regulating and soothing your feelings, so you don't get swept away. Conscious participation with your changing thoughts and emotions, challenge, compassion, leaning into what you aren't saying, reflecting, practising self-care, working on your relationships and intimacy – all what we have termed 'everyday mental maintenance' – ultimately allows you to grow.

JODIE'S STORY

I'm Jodie, the founder of Self Space. I was born in a small village in East Sussex in 1978; most of my peers were taught that feelings were for softies, drinking to excess regularly was normal and pulling yourself together and getting on with it was the only way. I watched emotional dysfunction and conflict destroy roots within my family; I have been trying to make sense of those upturned roots ever since. I was an apprentice in life, in a system that did not have the infrastructure, tools, manual or leader to show us how to make sense of being. Communication, emotions and acknowledgement of vulnerability were in dark recess for the entirety of my childhood. There just wasn't space under the thick blanket of financial uncertainty, promiscuity and booze for feelings, let alone to have any emotional needs understood or met. At times it felt paralysing, like I couldn't even begin to believe there might be a different way. But, like my siblings, I was propelled forward by the force of so much systemic libido and life drive – survival instincts at their best. So much laughter, so many traumas survived and celebrated, so many fried potato peelings with garlic salt, so much tenacity and vibrancy. So much love. I fully believe that love in itself is not an answer, but it definitely helps.

From those foundations I emerged at the core with an enormous capacity to process and bear witness to difficult things, to stand alongside others in their pain and confusion without needing to rush them on. I held on to the belief that there is always the potential for change, coupled with an abundance of curiosity: 'What can I make sense of here?', 'What can I understand and what can't I?', 'Can we take these roots and grow something new?'

What a monumental day it was when I walked away from my growing career as a TV presenter (which made me utterly miserable) to train as a therapist. I was not specific about the why at the time; I just knew I had to stop presenting and begin *feeling*. I had to visit the opposite pole to the one I was inhabiting.

I find myself returning over and over to that gut feeling that propelled me to become a therapist – that familiar place of knowing in the therapy room, the knife-edge of despair and hope, that junction between paralysis and movement. My own experience of it allows me to stand with my clients when needed, as they begin to understand what tools they have and what path they are taking.

Please know that, as you read this, I walk alongside you too, as I continue to try to work myself out, struggling often to make sense of it all. I show up here as a parent, a friend, a daughter, a wife, a niece and a sibling, an entrepreneur and a therapist, in the hope of being, at best, good enough. I readily use the tools we'll share in this book to help me navigate and stay on track. I don't believe we do, or indeed should, have it all together all of the time. We have to apply ourselves to learning, to equipping ourselves better for life's ups and downs. I hope that, once you've read this book, you'll feel more confident as you stand in the eye of everyday storms, that you have a little of what you need to keep you standing and that you are armed with some tools to help you grow.

CHANCE'S STORY

I'm Chance. I grew up in the north-east of England in a place called Hartlepool, a town stranded on its own lonely spit of sea-battered rock, out of the loop, at the end of the road with its back turned to the rest of the world. I was brought up by my nan and an army of north-eastern women, aunties and cousins. At the time of my birth, both my parents were caught up in substance addictions. At the age of eight my dad had died of an overdose, and when I was 25, my mum died under the same circumstances. Generations of alcoholism, addiction and poverty meant that there was no vocabulary I could draw from to put words to my internal world, no words for feelings and inner thoughts – only anger, grit, numbing and cutting off.

There was a peculiar loneliness growing up in a house where nobody knew how you felt; conversations would happen behind closed kitchen doors, there were regular ruptures and infrequent repairs, and nobody would talk about their feelings. But I always had a pull towards a deeper understanding of what was going on around me and inside me. I carried this curiosity with me within my own psychoanalysis. I started wanting to know more about myself, particularly the hidden parts, so nothing was left festering behind closed doors. Even after years of therapy, and robust and extensive therapy training, I find myself left with more questions than answers. I think this is the beauty of the work – it is unending, not quite reaching a finish line, but always close, always becoming and unbecoming.

I started my career as a therapist within addiction centres and '12 Step'-based recovery programmes across London. I worked with unaccompanied minor refugees and asylum seekers, and within pupil referral units before moving into adult mental health. I sighed with relief when I met Jodie. Finally, someone down in the trenches with clients and not on a pedestal – someone willing to get stuck in and do something about the increasingly stagnant field of therapy and how it is accessed.

At Self Space, in some way, we carry these experiences with us as founders. We have created a service focused on prevention, not reaction – a space where good conversations can take place with qualified people and where mental maintenance can happen in an everyday way. This book has the intention of extending this ethos outside of the therapy room, of creating a micro-experience of therapy in the pages that follow. A place where you may find yourself or your loved ones, where you might make clear parallels between our words and your life, in the same way that the therapy room is a mini-ecosystem for the wider world – a rehearsal room to play things out before taking them to the main stage. This book is exactly that – a place to play around with ideas about yourself.

What we have between us and our team of therapists are thousands of hours in the therapy room, with the most incredible and intimate lens into how people think, feel and behave. Because of that privilege, we can share with confidence the things that we hear over and over again that make a positive impact. We can share, here, ways of making your self-enquiry less daunting and offer up some tools to help you make more sense of yourself.

How to Use This Book

To grow, you will need to face, experience and process the shit that life throws at you. That is inevitable. In preparation, and to fortify your resources, this book is a guide to building stamina, so that you have the chance to grow though what you go through. See it as an encouragement towards self-compassion, curiosity, wisdom, self-awareness and buoyancy that we hope will support you when you need it most.

In writing this book, our aim is to encourage you to embrace your messiness and to feel more connected to and less ashamed of your human complexities. We will support you with some of our clinical wisdom, stories of ourselves and others (though we have made every effort to disguise the identities of our patients), and tips and ideas for mental maintenance. We also want to illustrate that *none* of us has all our shit together – we are all struggling, uncertain and confused at times, and that is more than OK. (Wherever we have used the term 'parent', we mean it to refer to both parent and carer.)

We take you through those bigger emotions such as grief, loss, anxiety, depression, fear, joy, hope and love, as well as exploring the impact of your past, the challenges of your present, the worries and hopes for your future. We look at the complexities of change and the life milestones you might face, such as parenting, separation and divorce, the death of a loved one, or new starts and endings, among others. But, crucially, we want you to come away with some suggestions and a safe place to turn to within these pages when life feels confusing or hard. We want to give a voice to all of us who are struggling and fearful, and offer the tools you can use to grow and embrace positive change.

Our experience of being equipped to grow through challenges means practising self-care little and often, daily – what we term 'everyday mental maintenance'. We have to work at good mental health. It would be pretty remarkable if we could promise that this book will help you to feel better quickly or achieve a constant state of happiness. Instead, like therapy, it offers a combination of empathy and challenge, both a gentle hand and a kick up the arse.

We aren't hoping for a cult-like belief in our words and this isn't a prescription for happiness ever after. We invite you to take what speaks to you from this book, challenge yourself where you find resistance and ignore what you don't like.

We know how much courage it takes to begin, because we've been there too. Thanks for trusting in us and the process, and – we hope – inviting in something new. But mostly, let's take a moment of gratitude for yourselves for starting.

TIME FOR REFLECTION

Find a notebook that doesn't have your to-do list in and a pen to keep at your side. Turn off your notifications, unclench your jaw, unknit your brow and relax your shoulders. Breathe in for four and out for four and ask yourself:

» Why did I pick up this book?

» What is my hope for myself right now?

» Where is it that I begin today?

» How am I really?

You can begin to write down the answers to these questions now, if you like, but as you go through the book, things will inevitably become clearer. Take note of the changes in your answers too – they can be different on different days.

Use this notebook to jot down things throughout the book that speak to you, in moments of reflection. We have included these 'Time for Reflection' boxes throughout, as well as journal prompts that you might like to try too.

And so, we find ourselves together here on the cusp of something new: two therapists debunking the myth of the untroubled therapist. The pages in this book hold hope for something different, some new understanding of yourself or of others. Perhaps you have opened this book with some or no expectations. Perhaps you've landed here alone, afraid, confused, hopeful, excited, in search of meaning. However you are, however you're feeling, you are here and so are we. We know that the thing that binds us here at the start of the book is our humanness. We are all in this together, perfectly imperfect, none of us immune to life's challenges. We can't promise miracle fixes, but we hope you will find some light-bulb moments or feel a hand on yours as we journey together. Whatever you find, we are glad to be here with you.

PART 1

The Basis of Your Mental Health

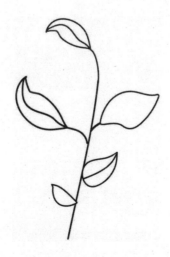

As we delve into the first section of this book, we intend to lay to rest any confusion or uncertainty you might have about the often misused terms associated with mental health. Understanding what is actually meant by 'mental health' will help you move towards some acceptance that we all have it, rather than the common misconception that mental health or mental ill health only belongs to some people, for example people with diagnosed 'mental health conditions'. We have a predisposition to misunderstanding, pathologising terms associated with mental health. Mental health language is still both overused yet under-understood, often provoking fear and shame, particularly in the UK where talking, thinking and education around mental health has historically only been connected to illness. Understanding and feeling educated about mental health terms can give you the personal power to begin deeper discovery, giving you words to wrap around what might feel, at times, impossible to articulate.

We also aim to give you the ammunition to shed some of those unhelpful generalisations that are commonly bandied around. Do you recognise any of these?

» If you feel a bit down, then there's something wrong with you that needs to be fixed.

» If you're not doing what everyone else is doing, you're not doing enough.

» If you don't feel grateful all the time, you're not a good person.

» Happiness should be a permanent state.

» You should only feel positive feelings.

» You are lucky to have your life, your parents, your partner, your job, and you should be grateful.

» Only if you are deemed clinically unwell will you struggle with your mental health.

» Happiness should shine out of your face like sunbeams all the time.

None of these expectations and pressures are realistic or useful for your well-being. Our intention is to extend some compassion to the universally shared messiness of being human and more motivation to *feel* your feelings and be less afraid of them. Feelings are a vital feedback system to our deeper selves and if we aren't able to listen and try to understand them, who will?

We also hope to dispel any reservations you might have about how you ended up here on these pages. It is not fate that you respond to, experience and inhabit the world around you as you do – your early experiences are pivotal in directing the human you are today. Horrid as it can sometimes be, there is so much merit in reflecting the past in order to shine a little light into the future. Let's do this, shall we?

Chapter 1

What is 'Mental Health'?

Often, the terms 'mental health', 'mental well-being' and 'mental illness' are used interchangeably in a way that suggests they share the same meaning, but the three are not synonymous. Let's look at what they mean, along with other key terms you might encounter:

Mental health is an essential and integral part of our health. Up until now, mental health has been thought about in terms of there being an absence of mental illness or mental disorders. It is often referred to as a purely positive state of being, marked by feelings of happiness and a sense of mastery over one's life. But it is much more than being happy, being in control and being without illness. When we are in good mental health, we can make the most of our potential. We feel as if we are thriving and can cope with what life throws at us. We can play a full part in our relationships, workplace and community. With good mental health, we can live our lives as close as is possible to the way we want to. Think of mental health as a 'continuum' with mental illness at one end and mental well-being at the other.

Mental illness refers to specific signs and symptoms that cause significant and persistent emotional distress. It affects how we feel, think, behave, cope, process information, make decisions and engage in our interpersonal relationships. The presence of such signs and symptoms indicates mental health disorders, such as anxiety disorders, depression, eating disorders, addictive behaviours and personality disorders. Approximately one in four of us in the UK will experience mental illness each year. Factors like poverty, genetics, biochemistry, childhood trauma, injustice, chronic stress or ongoing physical illness make it more likely that we will develop mental illness, but any of us can experience it. More often than not, people wait until this point before seeking therapy or support.

Mental well-being is what we experience if we are at the 'good mental health' end of the continuum. Here we are in tune with our thoughts and feelings. We can deal with and cope with change. We can solve problems and make decisions, and be flexible in the face of adversity. We can do things that we consider important and worthwhile. We can communicate our needs clearly, build strong relationships and understand ourselves and the world around us. We can hold the capacity for empathy, not only towards others but towards ourselves.

Mental maintenance is a term and practice that we devised to support our clients to move towards, remain in, or stay as close as they can to, a place of sustainable mental well-being. It isn't very complicated in its essence, but it's really powerful in practice.

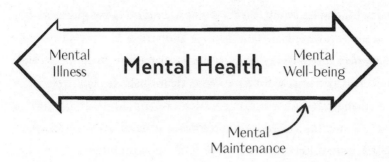

Mental health continuum

Everyday Mental Maintenance

We are sure you are all familiar with the term 'step-by-step' and have some experience of its positive relevance and helpfulness in your life (we don't always apply it to things we should and Jodie still tries to do all her Christmas shopping in a day, but . . .). Most of us learnt the idea of building things up incrementally at school with, say, reading and maths, and now understand it in relation to saving money, fitness, training pets, learning a new skill, and so on. We understand that we don't usually nail things in one go and that sometimes the boring, monotonous, step-by-step approach is the best way to build a solid foundation.

We suspect that you also recognise the importance of maintenance and repair on your property, car, bike, hair . . . You understand what helps to maintain your physical health, daily, monthly, yearly, and what it means to do the repetitive jobs at home and work that keep things running smoothly. Well, it's not surprising then that when we apply the same step-by-step approach and consistent maintenance to our mental health practices, we get good results.

Mental maintenance is a concept we have developed over our years of practice and one that we keep close to the ethos of our mission at Self Space. We see the results in the work we do with clients, the impact of how we educate our corporate partners and the value we spread across the team, always championing a realistic, bite-sized, proactive, 'do the work' relationship with our mental health.

Not all of us will experience a mental illness, but each of us human, vulnerable, fragile beings will, at some point, face challenges when it comes to our mental health. Every now and then it will be knocked off-kilter. A series of sleepless nights, growing pressures at work, being in touch with something painful from our childhood, anxieties about our health, relationships or finances, periods of loneliness, experiences of discrimination and stigma, times of turbulent change, the death of someone we love, the news, the weather, our political landscape, an argument, a break-up, a heartbreak, a holding of an unspoken truth . . . these are just some of the things that can make us feel out of whack. Considering how often we face these challenges in our daily lives, it really serves us to practise 'mental maintenance'.

In our culture we want quick fixes for things and we want them yesterday. When it comes to problem-solving, efficiency and instant gratification, we are pretty spoilt. We have an incredibly vast amount of immediately accessible stimuli to alleviate feelings, emotions or sensations that we might find difficult or satisfying: Tired? Get a coffee. Lonely? Head to the dating apps, social media or WhatsApp. Hungry? Order some food. Late and no taxis? Uber. Bored? Netflix or Asos.

When it comes to mental maintenance, however, quick fixes are less likely (and don't trust anyone who tells you otherwise!). Exploring our inner worlds and our emotions in a mindful, focused way, without distractions, can be uncomfortable. But know that discomfort is part of the process and that growth happens in the tears, anger, pain, frustrations, uncertainty and questioning. Know that we are here with you, accepting it all without judgement, and that we are doing the same ourselves.

THE BRAVE FACE

Each of us is full of self-doubt, fear, anxiety and confusion, but the brave, 'filtered' face has been so widely adopted. The brave face has made it easy to assume that everyone else is doing better than us. We think we are weird because we meet such edited versions of each other. However, most of the time, we have no idea what people are really experiencing or feeling. We have no idea how much someone has had to pull themselves together each morning.

Everyday mental maintenance challenges us to spare ourselves the burden of feeling alone in our struggles. It is about being OK with not feeling OK. By engaging in everyday mental maintenance, we can dissolve the need to be perfect and instead aim for 'good enough', allowing ourselves the space to fail and not hate ourselves for it. It is about treating ourselves as we would treat our best friend – with compassion and curiosity – in order to grow. It means not just reacting to mental illness, but taking a proactive approach to looking after our mental health and striving for mental well-being all year round. And in this case, it means us journeying together for a little while as we try to accept and understand the complexities we face. We are going to look at that in the next chapter.

Chapter 2

We're All a Bit Messy

How do you feel about the complexities of your feelings? Do you think of yourself as messy at times? If you do, what does that bring up for you? Are you quick to judge, admonish or tell yourself off? Do you distract, try to organise or banish what might feel too messy to sit with and process? What happens when you avoid what you don't want to see or explore? Are you left feeling out of sorts, a bit all over the place, not quite yourself?

Maybe you behave in ways which are actually depleting and exhausting, all in a bid to avoid what feels too messy. When we feel disturbance in our inner worlds but don't tend to it, it's like leaving something unsaid – we can feel incomplete, undone, not fully ourselves. A denial of our complexities gives us a deep-down sense of pretending, of being inauthentic somehow, so we feel off-kilter.

If we sit in a dark room with our hands over our ears because we are afraid, we can't see or hear what is in front of us. We might find that comforting (the controlling aspect of our psyche – the human mind, both conscious and unconscious – says, 'I am in charge here, my not seeing/hearing is a choice'), but ultimately we are disallowing ourselves the experience of anything other than fear. We do not really feel safe. We might be able to convince ourselves that we do, but it's a sort of pretend 'safe'. We create a suspended reality for ourselves. Yet, deep inside, we have a sense that we will need to open our eyes if we want to move from where we are. Staying in the room might be comfortable enough for a little while, but it will become properly boring soon. Somehow we know there is another side to our eye-opening, even if it feels very, very distant. Yes, we might well be gobbled up by a giant, man-eating monster, but most likely not. Most likely we'll locate the door and be able to leave. We might have to come back for socks or whatever, but next time it'll be less scary.

It's the same with our feelings: if we hide from them, we will not be able to feel them properly. If we can't feel them properly in all their often messy glory, we will not be able to move on from the place we are static in. We will not be able to grow. We might have a sense of moving through the motions of life on the outside – houses, jobs, birthdays . . . but we will not be living into the corners of ourselves. We'll feel off, not great, and our mental health will suffer as a result.

Don't Try to 'Marie Kondo' Your Feelings

I (Chance) was about three episodes into Netflix's *Tidying Up with Marie Kondo* when I found myself thinking: wouldn't my life be better if, when I opened my wardrobe, I didn't have unironed clothes half hanging on hangers and, instead, my clothes were all organised from dark to light, left to right, smart to casual? Wouldn't it be better if my sock drawer was arranged by colour gradient so that every time I opened it, I too would beam with serene joy at the rainbow it created – just like Marie Kondo? Creating this urge is the kind of thing Marie Kondo is incredibly skilled at. She excels at making what was previously seen as ordinary and laborious, attractive and exciting. She promises a framework that we can follow that allows us to not only optimise our home but *ourselves*. By following her trademark method, which essentially has two parts – discarding and sorting – we can create a world in which everything around us 'sparks joy'.

I was all-in. Who doesn't want everything around them to spark joy? Kondo tapped into something deep in my psyche (and the collective psyche of the millions of others who have watched her show and bought her book – that potent allure of organising that offers us the illusion of *control*. Human beings crave order, predictability and familiarity. From a survival perspective, predictability allows us to plan and better protect ourselves from potential threats. When things are uncertain, uncomfortable and outside our control, we seek out ways to reduce feelings of discomfort or helplessness and turn to things that distract us and help self-soothe, like cleaning and tidying. The opposite of messiness.

I told myself there was a healthiness in using cleaning to clear my mind, gain perspective and take a break from ruminating thoughts. It got my endorphins going and my blood pumping. I decluttered my space and it left me feeling somewhat accomplished and confident that I could take on other tasks.

But after conversations with my therapist, I quickly noticed that when we would get out the metaphorical scales that determined how much of what I was doing was healthy and how much of it was 'avoidant', they would constantly tip towards avoidant. I was cleaning to *avoid* internal discomfort: anxiety, worry and stress. And because it had brought about temporary relief, I found myself compelled to use the same technique every time an uncomfortable emotion would surface. But every time I stopped cleaning or started to mess up my newly organised space, the discomfort, anxiety, worry and stress would rebound even stronger than before. This is because I was teaching myself that I was unable to handle important feelings – that they were just too uncomfortable – so, to feel better, I just needed to avoid them. I was trying to control my messiness.

Our current culture pressures us into believing that if we are not happy, then surely there must be something wrong. So many self-help books promote the benefits of positive attitudes, positive vibes, positive thinking and positive habits. Many of them label sadness, anger, boredom, loneliness and grief as 'problems' or 'negative' emotions that need to be kept at bay, fixed or thought (sometimes fought) our way out of. So when challenging emotions leave us feeling heavy or uncomfortable, we tend to rush to our emotional exits in pursuit of distraction, quick relief and more joy or positivity.

Given that the majority of Western medicine is built upon the notion of eliminating pain, getting rid of it as soon as it shows up, it is not surprising that most of us approach the pain caused by our emotions in much the same way. While treating chronic pain and physical illness in this way may make the lives of sufferers more bearable, when we approach emotional pain in the same way, it is not healing. Instead, it robs our feelings of their potential to *teach us something* or to guide us in some important way.

What Lobsters Can Teach Us About Growth

Sadness, anger, boredom, loneliness and grief: we often treat them as unwanted guests that we want rid of as quickly as possible. Strong or challenging emotions are often signals for growth; we only need to look at lobsters to see how growth comes through adversity. When a lobster's shell becomes too rigid and confining, it begins to feel uncomfortable and under pressure. At this point, the lobster retreats somewhere safe, casts off its shell and releases the new one growing beneath. As this shell grows, it too gets uncomfortable and the lobster repeats the same process. The inducement for the lobster to grow is the very fact that it feels uncomfortable.

If lobsters had smartphones, Netflix or wine they would never cast off their shell and grow – they would be stuck in an endless loop of distraction. Humans can get stuck in this endless pursuit of quick relief or positivity. We seek out more of the 'neat, good' feelings (pleasure, excitement, love, happiness) and avoid the 'messy, bad' ones (sadness, anger, boredom, loneliness, grief, anxiety) at all costs. This, right here, is the source of a vast amount of our emotional struggles. It leaves us limited in the belief that because an emotion feels bad or messy, it *is* bad or messy.

The reality is that, when it comes to our emotional world, *we are all a bit messy*. Feelings and emotions don't live in tidy, labelled boxes making themselves known clearly. They get confused, they disguise themselves behaviourally as one thing when they are really something else. Feelings often live in a melting pot, blending into each other, confusing us and others around us, gathering energy from what they collide with. They burst out of our mouths, bodies, thoughts and behaviours in the hope of being seen and understood. They very rarely come in ways we can clearly understand: bar toilets are full of tears and feelings that can't quite be articulated; celebration parties are loaded with feelings which contribute to the reticent, jealous toast; baby showers are tinged with no-shows, and weddings with anger.

All of this can leave you with feelings of being overexposed, unprepared somehow for what's happening to you, without control over what it is you are doing or saying, why you are doing it or what your intentions are. This makes us feel off-balance, out of control, messy, and then we can feel as we have given too much of ourselves away. All of this contributes to feelings of shame and self-betrayal, which aren't very nice or productive – these feelings can also lead to further self-betrayal to block them out, and even disordered drinking, drug use, spending, sex . . . When you do not fully explore your complexities and open your arms and eyes to your messy feelings, you will not have mastery over how they live in the world.

We Are All a Beautiful Mess

It's fair to say that 'messy' as a concept is rarely celebrated. We don't like to think of ourselves as messy; there is something disordered, unpredictable and uncontained about it. It is understood most widely as a way of describing something that's confusing and difficult to deal with. We might find it talked about in the context of people's homes, cupboards or hair. Or maybe in the aftermath of a night out, a party, a divorce or a project that's all over the place. We do not look kindly on messy, drunk celebrities falling out of taxis or tangle-haired people on the train wearing smudged make-up. We prefer to fiercely disassociate with the messy narrative as having nothing to do with us. Court cases are full of mess, with a judge and jury trying to tidy up and make sense of what is presented to them.

So powerful is our negative association of 'messy' and messy emotions, that we will often do anything not to take responsibility or ownership over our messy selves. The shame, fear and self-judgement we can feel about getting it wrong, messing it up, being, feeling and behaving a bit shittily when we go through hard times, can lead us to expensive acts of 'disownership', which can be costly for our well-being and feelings of authenticity. We would rather adopt a stiff upper lip, keeping up appearances, than say, 'I am behaving dreadfully, I don't feel so good and I'm not sure what's going on. Can we talk it through?'

The world over, people who appear to have it all together (neat, tidy, linear lifelines) are perceived as doing better, as being more successful and somehow more acceptable than those who don't. Britney Spears is a prime example of how we treat and admonish emotional messiness. She has been judged, hounded and punished in various ways for what is presented to us as her lack of personal and emotional neatness, her lack of 'having it all together'. She's often referred to as 'a mess'. Yet isn't she really a wonderful, truthful example of how we all feel and behave sometimes? When she arrives on her social channels just as she is – vulnerable, uncertain, unpresentable – isn't she so deeply relatable? The bandwagon everyone jumped on initially was to vilify her; we got entrenched in shame and a sort of icky discomfort. As we reject Britney's humanness, we are actually trying to expel what is deeply complex, vulnerable, disordered and shameful in ourselves. We reject her messiness by proxy as we also reject our own. Maybe this makes us feel accomplished somehow. Superior.

TIME FOR REFLECTION

» Do you often compare yourself to others?
» Do you judge your own difficult, complex, messy emotions against others' order/togetherness?
» Do you label your own success or failure based on what you perceive as the difference between yourself and others?

This black-and-white thinking and often contempt for that which cannot be easily ordered, sorted out or understood, can be at best unhelpful and at worse condemning and derailing. A client referred to this cycle of comparing his own mental health against others as 'I do my own head in – it's like a competition I'll never win. I am always in a total state compared to everyone else and I feel I just have to pretend I'm like them, with it all sorted.' We commonly want to brush the mess under the carpet in an attempt to hide it, disallowing us the often rich experience of deeper investigation into its contents, ultimately denying ourselves the magic that might be found within the mess if we were able to take some ownership.

I (Jodie) remember, in the early days of parenthood, receiving a voice message from a friend who I'd spent the day with. Both our daughters were under two and it was a stressful, lonely, boring and often overwhelming parenting period. Her message, 'Thanks for a lovely day, so nice to get the kids together, glad to see we're both loving it all', ended with her unintentionally not disconnecting the phone and capturing her shouting 'Will you just stop? Your crying is driving me loopy!' to a screaming toddler. To which I could fully relate and empathise. The polarity between what she said/showed me and what she was really feeling was vast. Both of us wore the mask of 'having it all together' so well that we denied ourselves the opportunity for being together as we really were. Did I think less of my friend? No. Did I feel connected to her experience? Yes . . . and I felt relief that I wasn't the only one.

We would much prefer to show our struggling selves to the world in any different way than we actually are, widening the gap between what we feel and what we show. We jump to quick exits of displacement, rejection, repression or denial when what we are faced with is not neat or simply understood. This is exactly why social media is such a challenge to our emotions. When we see posts that appear authentic, how much are we really seeing? Would we see washing stuffed in corners and unmade beds in the perfect lifestyle shot? Would we see junk food wrappers in the bin on the seven-day juice diet feeds? How many of your own posts have you curated, even just a little, to hide yourself?

'MESSY CAN LEAVE THE TABLE'
(AND OTHER UNHELPFUL STUFF WE GOT TAUGHT)

So how did we get into this segregated, unhelpful thinking about our emotions? How did we get to a place where some of us were told our feelings weren't valid, that we were too messy, too complex, too different? That unless we conformed, we would not be allowed, let alone invited, to sit with those who did and could conform?

One reason might be that, from an early age, it is ingrained into many of us that messiness, disorder, different beliefs and values, or behaviours that don't follow family norms, are an indication that we are not doing well, that we are below par, that we are flawed. From early on, we are taught that 'good' and 'acceptable' behaviour is often neat, contained, the same as 'everyone else'. We are praised for tidying up, washing our hands, wiping away our tears, pulling ourselves together, closing the door on temper tantrums, cleaning our plates, wiping our noses, being seen and not heard, conforming to social norms. We see this so often in the therapy room – as children, we are slowly socialised towards demanding less of others with our emotions.

We have been discouraged away from our mess in overt and subtle ways since birth. It is no wonder, then, that when we encounter our very human emotional messiness, we are often terrified, embarrassed and shamed into silence. We are constantly doing our best to appear tidy and together, cohesive to the expectations of others, both within our families and the wider world.

TIME FOR REFLECTION

» What relationship do you have with your own messiness, your own often unfathomable emotional responses?

» How might these have been shaped?

» How have your own views around the messier, less palatable parts of yourself been formed?

» What do you remember about how your caregivers responded to your emotions when you were young?

» If you think about 'messiness', are you transported back to your family and your experiences within your family?

Most damaging opinions are formed, not by how you experienced your own mess, but by how others in caregiving or authoritative roles responded to it and how that made you feel. We can see it happening all around us: tutting on buses when children cry too much; parents/carers feeling uncomfortable and trying to hush the child; children being sent out of the classroom when emotions run too high and being told to calm down. Or a colleague being shot down at a board meeting if they become 'too emotional'; everyone nodding in support of the prosecutor, feeling delighted at the emerging conflict.

How was mess viewed in your family home – both actual mess and emotional mess? Were you punished if you didn't tidy your room, were you blackballed if you became too emotional, labelled the 'drama queen' or the 'too sensitive one'. Did you bear witness to people being talked about with repulsion and pity: 'look at him, such a mess'? If you felt too overwhelmed to get up, were you called lazy? If you felt too full of emotion to eat, were you called fussy? If you felt so empty that you couldn't stop eating, were you called greedy, or were others around you labelled in this way? If you were moody, if you were jealous, if you were angry, were you ignored or grounded/kept in (the opposite of what anger needs, which is space and light and energy)?

Emotions can be dismissed vehemently within families, which is damaging and silencing. They can also be dismissed and minimised more subtly – even accidentally – when attention or focus isn't being paid or there is low emotional intelligence in the family. Were you cheered up when you felt miserable or sent out to do exercise for moping around? Maybe you were denied your experience by being told you were lying, exaggerating or making it up. When we are invalidated, even in a small way, we are being shown that our feelings don't matter, which can be distressing and can impact on how we relate to our feelings in the future. It is important to note here that being agreed with isn't the same as being validated; not everyone will agree with what you are feeling, but being invalidated and ushered away from your feelings can be detrimental to your mental health. Did you ever hear any of these invalidating terms in your family?

» 'You're too sensitive.'
» 'Come on, it wasn't that bad.'
» 'You always take things too personally.'

» 'You'll get over it.'

» 'Just let it go.'

» 'You're strong, you're better/bigger than this.'

» 'It could be worse/you don't have it as bad as X.'

» 'Everything happens for a reason.'

» 'I know exactly how you feel/I feel the same.'

» 'You shouldn't be angry/be upset/cry.'

» 'Pull yourself together.'

» 'You make a big deal out of everything.'

» 'That didn't happen/you imagine things/you aren't in the real world.'

» 'Stop making things up.'

» 'You're overreacting.'

» 'You probably misunderstood.'

» 'Shut up/stop crying.'

Or did you receive non-verbal reactions to your emotions, such as eye-rolling, being ignored or talked over, playing on devices, mimicking you, copying you, people walking away from you?

JOURNAL PROMPT

Take a minute to note down any behaviours and words which felt invalidating to you. Feel free to add any we've missed. This is not by way of persecuting those around you, but a moment of compassion for what's gone before. Reflect on how it may still be impacting how you feel about your feelings and how you treat them.

We have been steered away from enquiry and into categorising behaviour as 'good' and 'bad' without even knowing it. Your opinion-forming and your own self-judgement will have been based formatively on what was happening around you and how others judged, spoke about or treated emotional messiness. All of this causes us to repress feelings and banish behaviours that communicate feelings by enforcing them into repression. Most of us have been taught: Stay tidy, or else.

I (Jodie) worked with Lucy (37) over the course of a year. She came to see me because she was struggling with her relationship of four years and felt she wasn't able to let her partner into her inner world. This was making her feel alone and often angry at him. In our eighth session she told me that after the separation of her mum and dad when she was seven years old and her father leaving the family home, she was told not to speak about, have contact with or look at pictures of him. She recalled that any trace of him was removed from the family home – it was as if he had 'just vanished'. If Lucy expressed any emotions about missing him, or sadness, confusion or anger over the loss of him from her life, she was sent to her room. She was not allowed to ask questions about him or share memories. This left her with an enormous amount of complicated feelings with nowhere to go to process them. She made up stories about him and turned him into a film character in her mind as a way of coping.

Lucy had no way to process the very complicated things she was feeling about a daddy she loved who had suddenly disappeared. She had no point of reference to anchor her emotions to, no place to ask questions, speak her feelings or even just be sad. It is not until years later, after his death, as we sit face-to-face in the therapy room, that we invite it all in – everything she was not allowed or encouraged to share back then, the feelings which she now recognises as becoming distorted after years of being kept inside, emotions that have grown in power over time in the dark.

After her father's death, Lucy was given a box of things that were his, but she had not been able to look inside it. She brought this to the therapy room and we opened it together. She had a chance to piece together what she now knows about him, and we thought about the many things she would like to have asked him or said. Her curiosities, sadness and hopes, her memories and feelings are invited in. Over the course of our sessions, as she speaks those unspoken words from years ago, she keeps looking at me, checking she's not in trouble, checking I'm not going to ask her to leave or, worse, leave her. The more she spoke her feelings out loud, the more she realised how valid they all were, how OK it was for her to have felt them – then and now – and we were able to reach out to her with compassion and understanding. She had harboured so much shame for feeling her feelings, telling herself over the years that she should just have been able to make him vanish from her feeling world and, when she couldn't, she spent years punishing herself.

We decided that she'd share the contents of the box with her partner as a way of bridging the gap between them and giving him insight into her, developing intimacy.

This was a great building block for how they related in the future – she was able to identify her fear of letting him in as a protective measure against him also vanishing. She was able to share this with him and he met her in reassurance and understanding rather than the rigid and often fractious experiences that they had been having. We used the metaphor of the box over our future work and Lucy began to identify when she put things in a box inside of herself, judging and banishing complex feelings. I was able to encourage her to recognise when she did this and to do it less. With more consciousness, she began to reorientate her relationship to feel her feelings for the better.

I suspect what was really happening in this situation – and it is not uncommon in split families – is that her mother was terrified of her own complicated feelings about the situation. Any proximity to softness around it was too much for her to cope with, so for her own self-protection, she banished the father and her feelings away, unaware of the impact this would have on the children.

What if we approach our emotions in the same way as lobsters do their shells (see page 27)? Suppose we retreat to the safety of a quiet moment within ourselves, with a friend or with a therapist, and try to grow through what we go through. Suppose we sit with our difficult feelings for long enough for them to teach us what we need to know. Sooner or later, we will be able to cast them off and grow from them, rather than harbouring them in the dark.

JOURNAL PROMPT

Can you identify anything from your past that was not given space or light that you still carry today?

» How was it treated back then?
» How did that make you feel?
» What did you/it really need?
» Can you identify if and how it impacts your life now?
» Can you take a moment to extend some self-compassion and what would that sound or look like?

Looking at these difficult things encourages us to grow. It gives us a chance to take nutrients from what we have been through and it gives us confidence to identify and inhabit our challenging feelings, without combusting. The more we do this, the more we are reassured that our feelings are temporary. Our feelings and emotions give us a fuller sense of ourselves and the complexity involved in being human. It brings us closer to authenticity.

ALL VIBES WELCOME

This is an invitation to you to lay down the exhausting pressure to be constantly happy. To lay down the pressure to feel as though you have to have it figured out at all times. It is an invitation to shift your focus away from striving for perfection and, instead, step into flexibility, curiosity and compassionate self-enquiry.

In these pages, let's create space for new and more inclusive definitions of mental well-being, as free as possible from restrictive and invalidating statements like 'positive vibes only', 'everything happens for a reason', 'other people have it much worse' and 'you should be grateful for what you've got' – and as close as possible to how we experience life as human beings – sometimes beautiful, and at other times disgusting; sometimes calm, and at other times chaotic and seriously hard to navigate. Not just 'positive vibes' only – all vibes are allowed here.

Chapter 3

All the Feels

Tending effectively to emotional mess is determined by our ability to hold, experience and make space for it. The only way we can allow for movement in the way we feel is by becoming aware of our inner experience, embracing the mess and learning to befriend what is going on inside ourselves. It is knowing that there are no bad emotions. It is by allowing ourselves to *feel* (both heavy and light), without judgement, that we grow.

Feeling Shitty is Not a Sign That You're Doing Life Wrong

Difficult emotions are a part of being a fully feeling, messy and complex human being. It is in those spaces of uncertainty and discomfort that we really get to know our growing edges. There, holding the tension between the old and the new, at once vulnerable and resilient. If we don't allow ourselves the opportunity to grow, to take the risk of it, we can never really know our own potential. When we invalidate or judge our own emotions, we strip them of their ability to teach us. Have you ever said any of these things to yourself?

» 'I shouldn't feel this way.'
» 'Why can't I just stop it?'
» 'Get your shit together!'
» 'People have it worse off.'
» 'It's not that bad.'
» 'I just need to get over it.'

Sound familiar? These are all ways of invalidating how we feel. Everyone feels emotions. The problem is when we judge our emotions or refuse to feel them. When we suppress emotions, they don't go away; they only get stronger. Uncomfortable emotions, like sadness, hurt, anxiety, grief and anger, come to us as big, bright neon lights from the body and brain. They are signs that something is out of alignment in or around us – they don't happen because of some 'weakness' within us. What creates true emotional endurance and buoyancy is what we do and think when difficult feelings come to us.

What Am I Feeling?

Feelings are confusing. They don't show up with labels identifying what they are, with instruction manuals on how to best tend to them. They often arrive surrounded by other feelings, dressed up as something they are not, confusing us and making it harder for us to identify what we might be feeling – and subsequently what we might need to support ourselves. We might rush to identify what we are feeling, justifying the emotion to ourselves as appropriate to an event or thought and then leaving it there without pursuing it further. Without drilling a little deeper into what we are actually feeling, we can often rush ourselves into feeling better or *pretending* to feel better.

For example, you see a social media post or receive a message from a friend to say they have a great new job. This might prompt you to feel jealous, envious, cross or frustrated. You momentarily feel it and then brush over it, telling yourself you are a horrid person for feeling that way, pressuring yourself to instead reach out in celebration, offering congratulations perhaps, which is the expected thing to do. In doing so, you abandon yourself, leave yourself behind. You might find you feel brittle, upset or just a bit 'off' when you next see the friend. You might find ways of disliking the friend to put distance between you and them, finding it too hard to confront. As a consequence, you don't fully connect to the feeling that perhaps you are not confident enough – or feel you are not good enough – to look for a new job or realise your own potential.

TIME FOR REFLECTION

When you feel strong emotions, you can start by asking yourself these questions:

» What happened?

» What strong emotion am I experiencing?

» What are the sensations in my body telling me?

» What story am I telling myself (if any) about what it means to feel this way?

> » How can I purposefully allow myself to feel this emotion(s)?
> » Do I have to feel it alone?
> » What can I accept (however big or small) in what I'm feeling?
> » What has this emotion come to teach me?
> » What are the thoughts/beliefs that don't align with my values?

If you can allow difficult feelings to form fully-fledged, you can gather important information about yourself. Maybe you are dissatisfied, unfulfilled or feeling left behind – in doing so, you get a bit closer to what's really going on for you and what you might need. If you don't encourage yourself into more enquiry, you can sometimes become stuck where you are. You can't grow if you're stuck.

We discover much more about ourselves if we uncover our truest, often more vulnerable, emotions. If not, we might jump to the wrong conclusions about ourselves, based on incorrect information. For example, if you are angry because you have been lied to, yes, perhaps you are immediately angry, but you might also feel wounded, betrayed and vulnerable. Without delving into the deeper layer of intel, you might rush to treat your anger with a run, a vent or an argument, ignoring the other emotions that might need caring for in completely different ways.

FEELINGS IN DISGUISE

Feelings are able to disguise themselves very well. Sometimes they show up as familiar emotions or sometimes something totally different:

» Anger: dressed up as sadness, resentment or despair.
» Jealousy: dressed up as over-compliance or hate.
» Shame: dressed up as resentment or fear.
» Dependence: dressed up as independence.
» Hope: dressed up as anxiety.
» Shyness: dressed up as humour or confidence.
» Fear: dressed up as courage.
» Doubt: dressed up as absolute certainty.

These acts of disguise can make it particularly difficult for us to understand how we might support our feelings. How can we take care of something if we don't know what it is?! When you identify a feeling, take a moment to think about what your feelings might be, hidden away beneath the surface.

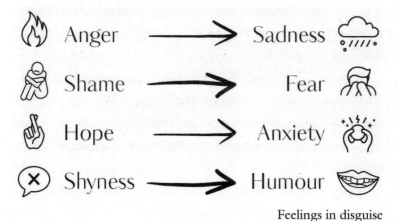

Feelings in disguise

The difference between sadness and depression

As therapists, we've met many people struggling with depression who thought they were just 'sad'. We have also met many people who were extremely sad and worried they might be depressed. Because we associate depression with its primary symptom of pervasive sadness, many of us struggle to tell the difference.

On the surface, sadness and depression are very similar. Both can make people feel alienated from their normal lives, and withdrawn from relationships and the world. But there is one categorical difference between depression and sadness: the sad person knows what they are sad about; the depressed person doesn't.

Sadness is a normal human emotion. We've all experienced it and we all will again. Sadness is usually triggered by a difficult, hurtful, challenging or disappointing event, experience or situation. Sad people can, without difficulty, tell us what is troubling them: 'I've lost my job', 'I've been hurt by someone I love', 'I've been let down', 'Someone I love has died'. We tend to feel sad about *something*. This also means that when that something changes, when our emotional hurt fades, when we've adjusted or processed a loss or disappointment, our sadness gets lighter.

A depressed person often feels sad about *everything*. They can't conclusively put a finger on what's wrong. Depression affects our thinking, emotions, perceptions and behaviours in pervasive and chronic ways. Depression does not necessarily require a difficult event or situation, a loss or a change of circumstance as a trigger. In fact, it often occurs in the absence of any such triggers. People's lives on paper might be totally fine – they would even say this is true – and yet they still feel horrible.

Depression is sadness that has forgotten 'why'. Forgotten because remembering might be too overwhelming and unmanageable. When it comes to the signs and symptoms that sadness has crossed over into depression, there are three areas of our well-being that are impacted:

1. **Psychological.** The psychological symptoms of depression include: continuous low mood or sadness; feeling hopeless and helpless; having low self-esteem; feeling tearful; feeling guilt-ridden; feeling irritable and intolerant of others; having no motivation or interest in things; finding it difficult to make decisions; not getting any enjoyment out of life; feeling anxious or worried; having suicidal thoughts or thoughts of harming yourself.
2. **Physical.** The physical symptoms of depression include: moving or speaking more slowly than usual; changes in appetite or weight; constipation; unexplained aches and pains; lack of energy; low sex drive (loss of libido); changes to menstrual cycle; disturbed sleep (for example, finding it difficult to fall asleep at night or waking up very early in the morning).
3. **Social.** The social symptoms of depression include: avoiding contact with friends; taking part in fewer social activities; neglecting your hobbies and interests; having difficulties in your home, work or family life.

Each of these symptoms often comes on gradually, so it can be difficult to know something is off-kilter. Almost half of us will suffer from depression at some point in our lives and many of us live and cope with depression without reaching out for support.

What about anxiety?

We can place anxiety on a long scale: at the low end is uneasiness and at the high end is paralysing terror. In between we find fear, social anxiety, agitation, dread and panic.

It can be said that anxiety is our fundamental state of being. As descendants of the savannah, we still carry the horrors of being trampled on and hunted by other species. Today, we live in incredibly busy environments, constantly bombarded with information that our brains are always left chasing to process. We rely on much of our comfort from other people whose needs and wishes don't always align with our own. We make big life decisions without really having the information we need to make them: a new job, a new flat in a new city, a new partner – we're often going off gut feeling, steering blind.

SIGNS YOU MIGHT BE FEELING ANXIOUS

Are you experiencing any of these? Sometimes, your feelings can be quite subtle or seem quite everyday to you, but they might be signs that you are anxious. Are you:

» Carrying physical tension?
» Skin-picking, nail-biting or foot-tapping?
» Increasing your alcohol intake?

» Procrastinating (putting things off)?
» Pre-crastinating (rushing through things to get them done)?
» Seeking distractions?
» Constantly planning ahead?
» Avoiding spontaneity?
» Seeking perfection?
» Finding it difficult to delegate to others/ask for help?

Of course, many of the things that cause us anxiety are part of being human and of living a full life. But there are times when anxiety can get in the way, impacting on the quality of your life; generalised anxiety disorder (GAD) can affect you both physically and mentally.

How do you know when everyday anxiety has crossed over into GAD? There are, again, three areas to consider:

1. **Psychological.** Psychological symptoms of GAD can cause a change in your behaviour and the way you think and feel about things. These include: restlessness; a sense of dread; feeling constantly 'on edge'; difficulty concentrating; irritability.

2. **Physical.** Physical symptoms of GAD include dizziness; tiredness; a noticeably strong, fast or irregular heartbeat (palpitations); muscle aches and tension; trembling or shaking; dry mouth; excessive sweating; shortness of breath; stomach ache; feeling sick; headaches; pins and needles; difficulty falling or staying asleep (insomnia).

3. **Social.** Your symptoms may cause you to withdraw from social contact, including seeing your family and friends, to avoid feelings of worry and dread. You may also find going to work difficult and stressful, and may take time off sick. These actions can make you worry even more about yourself and impact your self-esteem.

If you think this is you, that you are experiencing GAD or depression, then the first step is *acceptance*. There is no need – on top of everything else – to be anxious that you are anxious. There is no need to be guilty about feeling depressed. When it comes to anxiety or depression, we should spare ourselves the loneliness involved in 'just getting on with it'. We are far from the only ones who feel this way. Reach out to others, seek support.

THE FIGHT AGAINST FEELINGS

When it comes to the mass of confusing, complicated feelings we have going on as humans, is it any wonder that we would rather pretend we didn't have them? Our inclination to explore feelings and fully feel them, is thwarted by many things, such as our family values, our peers, our parents, other role models and social media.

We are amazing, incredible beings, full of so much intel about the world and the people around us. Yet, we find it so difficult to access our whole selves, preferring instead to repress less appealing feelings from our everyday repertoire. We would rather stay in the shell that is too small than try something new – not dissimilar to those awful old slippers or that broken lipstick we keep on using, which don't really do the job, but are known, and that feels more reassuring than something new. We become familiar with a set of emotions and stay with them regardless of whether they serve us well or not. *We stay comfortably uncomfortable.* This means many important, informative aspects of our emotional world remain unexplored. If we stay with what's comfortable, we rob ourselves of the chance to be in touch with the deeper aspects of ourselves.

This is really why both anxious and depressed feelings are so stubborn in not leaving – they are desperate to tell us something about ourselves. They really want some attention, like a child in the classroom who can't stop putting their hand up. The psyche is a smart ecosystem trying constantly to level itself out; it's just that sometimes we get in our own way.

When we avoid things constantly, they retain their elusive power and take control of the way we engage in the world and with others, often in ways we do not feel in charge of.

Things that make our emotions either get bigger or show up in places we don't expect:

» resisting them
» minimising them
» avoiding them
» judging them
» hating them
» ignoring them
» criticising them
» being afraid of them
» denying them
» defending against them

If we cannot bear to look,
we do not have the opportunity to grow.

TIME FOR REFLECTION

» When have you noticed yourself avoiding your emotions,
perhaps in some of the ways described above?

» How did you feel afterwards? Did those feelings get
bigger or did they shift towards numbness, depression,
anxiety or towards a different emotion entirely?

» Being honest with yourself, how do you think this may
have changed your behaviour and how you related
to the world at the time?

DEFENCE MECHANISMS

As much as we love to think about ourselves as rational, intellectual decision makers, most of the time we are driven by what
we *feel*, not what we *think*. Feelings can be utterly atrocious
and terrifying at times, so we do anything we can to avoid feeling them. Enter our trusty defence mechanisms: psychological
strategies and behaviours we use subconsciously to protect us
from anxiety or unbearable thoughts or feelings.

Defence mechanisms can be both outrageous and subtle;
they act as a way of protecting us from messy matter we may
not be equipped, prepared or able to process. Not all defence
mechanisms are totally unhelpful; many have helped us survive
painful, traumatic and upsetting events. However, when we
are not able to recognise *when* our defence mechanisms are in

action, we are left with emotional blind spots – we become a dot-to-dot with missing sections. Incomplete. We might find that our behaviour does not represent how we are really feeling. We might feel unseen, unheard and lonely, without the support we might have if we were able to be a little more in tune with ourselves.

TIME FOR REFLECTION

Can you notice the difference between what is comforting and what is a defence mechanism? Sometimes it's hard to tell the difference. Defensive feels avoidant and you might notice yourself moving away from what feels difficult. Comforting has an invitation to lean into a feeling, to feel the stress in all its glory while also finding ways to sooth yourself.

» Where do you go in times of stress?
» What do you do in times of stress?

Defence mechanisms can provide us with safety when we need it most and when we have no other options. Being able to identify what is defensive for you is incredibly useful to your growth and migration *away* from it. Do you recognise yourself in any of the following **defensive positions?**

Regression (retreating to a younger you)
When threatened, it's not uncommon for us to retreat or escape emotionally to a time or stage in our development when we

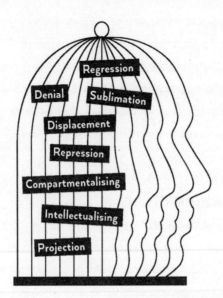

Defence mechanisms

were less burdened by our feelings. We see this frequently in young people – when they are faced with difficult or testing times, they will regress backwards to where they felt certain or safe, or to behaviours they associate with getting the attention they needed or craved. Sometimes the regression can be soothing and sometimes turbulent, depending on how well the stages were negotiated. You might find that your eating or sleeping patterns change or maybe you seek out the toys or activities that you cherished as a child. Thumb-sucking, nail-biting and fidgeting are common regressions we see in clients.

You may also forget, or be unable to do, more grown-up things you did with ease before, for example, ordering a drink at the bar or sorting out a train ticket might feel totally unmanageable. You might find you return to feeling uncertain, angry or self-conscious, much as you did as a teen. Or you might start to do silly things without considering the consequences.

Alex (49), separated, with two children, came to see me (Jodie). We worked together for 36 sessions. In our first session, he shared that he had recently begun collecting comics he read as a child. He would read some of the comics, but not all, and he felt he needed to order every edition. He found it comforting to be surrounded by the comics. Alex arrived expressing concern with his comic-buying, but less concerned with the recent separation from his wife, which he shared dismissively and quickly in session three. I was curious about the way he brushed this off, and the lack of discussion around her and his children. I began to press him gently on this aspect of his life over the coming sessions, pushing him to orientate himself in his current situation rather than the preoccupation with his comics (a past safe place).

   With some time, we were able to make space for his overwhelming distress at the loss of his relationship and he was able to make contact with his hopeless, despairing, grieving feelings and his longing for his children. In doing so, he was able to understand that the comic-buying was a desperate bid to try to return to a time when he felt safe as a child, to bring himself some comfort when he felt lost at sea. In understanding the function the comic-buying was playing, rather than Alex chastising himself over it, we were able to lean into the compassion and care that he really needed during this difficult time. In sharing the real-life challenges he was facing, his comic-buying decreased, as his needs were being more consciously met in our work. The comic-buying acted as a supportive defence mechanism when he needed it, but he knew in himself it wasn't solving his problems or supporting his growth. Alex knew something was not feeling good, but he needed some space to invite it all in and move beyond his defence mechanism.

Repression (locking it away)

Just because we tell ourselves we're over it, it doesn't mean we *are* over it. Banishing difficult feelings away into the depths of ourselves, ignoring them and brushing them off does not mean they are unfelt or unexpressed, even if we aren't consciously feeling them. In fact, when repressed, they often gather energy. You might find they powerfully drive your behaviours in ways you can't make sense of or that don't serve you well.

Repressed feelings have a way of making themselves known. We might then look for ways to distract ourselves from them, such as shopping, drinking, eating, substances or sex.

Projection

With feelings we find difficult, we might project them outwards as a way of avoiding owning or integrating them for ourselves. We split them off from ourselves and locate them in others. We do this with both the positive and the more challenging aspects of ourselves.

You might notice you detest a quality in a person or find some of their behaviour repulsive, yet on closer inspection, you understand it as something you share, something you would rather not know about yourself. A common example is a cheating spouse who suspects/accuses their partner of being unfaithful, or a bully who projects their feelings of vulnerability on to the victim and then punishes them for it. You might idealise or find someone's humour, creativity or style mega attractive, and think of your own self as not having these qualities, yet desire or admire them. We obsess over aspects of another rather than trying to actualise it in ourselves.

When we project ourselves we will often feel incongruent, not fully aligned with what we are saying or doing. We might feel guilty or out-of-sorts afterwards, but can't fully understand why. When someone projects on to us we might either identify with the projection (for example, the victim of the bully will most likely have feelings of being victimised or not good enough in other areas of their life), or we will feel angry, upset, in rejection of what is being projected on to us. This can cause friction in relationships if they aren't talked about. Some projections might go unnoticed by both parties.

TIME FOR REFLECTION

Can you notice when you are casting something out, throwing a projection?

» Start to take a mental note of when you feel you might be doing it, even if you aren't exactly sure what's happening.

» Notice when something you're saying doesn't quite fit with where you're sending it, or when what you're saying feels as if it might mean something else. Look for patterns.

Denial

Denial is one of the most common defence mechanisms. It occurs when we refuse to accept reality or facts. We block painful/difficult/complex/sad external events or circumstances from our minds so that we don't have to deal with the emotional impact. In other words, we avoid painful feelings or events and often adopt distraction methods (Netflix, wine, tidying up!).

Displacement

When we displace our feelings, we put/show/display them somewhere safe (or safer) so that we don't have to face them. This can be useful if it's conscious – for example, 'I'll take what I'm feeling to therapy to process' – but most often we are unconscious or perhaps partly unconscious that we are doing it.

You might notice that you direct strong, messy, less palatable emotions or frustrations towards a person or object that doesn't feel too threatening. This allows you to satisfy your need to react and express yourself, but you don't risk significant consequences.

A good example of displacement is being cross with your friend, partner or child because you had a rubbish day at work. None of these people is the target of your rage really, but reacting to them is less problematic than reacting to your boss or leaning into a much scarier conflict that might need to be addressed.

Displacement can be horrible in the aftermath, where we might feel guilt, shame and distress. We know that how we acted wasn't justified, but we don't fully understand why or what's happening and can't explain it. It can be terrifying to try to reclaim displaced feelings.

Sublimation (blocking off)

This is where we redirect our challenging feelings into something we feel we have mastery over. Grieving people might become marathon runners or yoga pros. We deploy our 'doing' function into overdrive as a way of containing and blocking off our more difficult feelings (hopelessness, overwhelm, sadness, jealousy, upset).

You might find that you launch heavily into work when things are feeling difficult internally. Work can feel, and sometimes is, a safe place to take refuge. It can feel safe with parameters you understand and are familiar with. But if we think about the image of our feelings being hidden under the many emails, work jobs and tasks we use to block them off, they don't disappear but instead become squashed and disjointed, possibly manifesting into resentment from overworking.

Blocking things off can sometimes be a useful way of managing or getting through as a coping mechanism, but there is only so much running away from our feelings we can do. We might notice our techniques become obsessive, all-consuming or disproportionate to their gain, but we can't stop. When we block off our feelings, they will most often find a way of escaping but with more gusto and less direction than if we had not blocked them off in the first place.

Blocked-off feelings also become incredibly jumbled. They have a chance to mingle with other blocked-off emotions, gaining in power and intensity. When we shut our feelings away or block them out of view, they can often become confusing or find a way of using a different channel to escape. For example, imagine you feel some hurt or pain around something someone says about you; perhaps it feels like a criticism, it makes you feel some sadness or upset as you cast it away, shut the door on it, put the brave face on. But where does it go? Not away but somewhere inside, where it might find residue of other criticisms and their pain, maybe from childhood, maybe from your first job, maybe from your partner. Shut away together, they might build in power, bursting out as uncontainable rage that feels disparate to the event – and maybe the bus driver who tutted when you dropped your pass gets the full brunt of those blocked-off feelings.

Compartmentalising (ordering)

Separating your life into neat sectors may feel like a way to keep control over those things that feel more uncontrollable. Imposing order on disorder without actually sorting through things can give us momentary relief.

We compartmentalise as a way of avoiding the anxiety and fear that can arise from the clash of contradictory values or emotions. For example, you might think of yourself as a nurturing, patient parent, but a precise authoritarian at work. You might find it hard for work colleagues to see you in your home life or catch wind of your softer side. You might perform the perfect daughter/son act in the company of your parents/carers but behave outrageously in your circle of friends. We often feel this strategy of hiding parts of ourselves is protecting us from conflict and exposure, and that it gives us certain power over how we are received or perceived, when, in fact, it places us on an island where we can often not be reached. These compartments full of feelings can create a divide away from intimacy, and no one sees a full and rounded view of how we are really doing. In addition, we become so used to being inauthentic that we can forget who we really are, resulting in feelings of shame if we are caught out as our other selves.

As with most defence mechanisms, there are times when compartmentalising can be useful and beneficial. For example, a paramedic may have a family that depends on them at home, but they must rush into life-threatening situations without hesitation to do their job and might need to compartmentalise to get through. When you need to finish an important project at work but know you also need to deal with a family conflict, compartmentalising might allow you to do both in a manageable way. Being able to compartmentalise those two realities allows you to perform under intense pressure. The same is true for soldiers, caring staff and those who work under huge amounts of trauma. But when we become used to repressing or compartmentalising certain aspects of ourselves, we do not show up anywhere as our authentic selves, which can be emotionally costly for a fulfilled life. If we do not find ways to merge the compartments, we can become distant from ourselves, disconnected and inauthentic.

Intellectualising

Sometimes when we are faced with really emotionally challenging life situations, we might try to gain mastery over them by removing emotion from what is happening – imposing our thinking function over feeling because it feels safer or more known to us, less messy. We move towards reason, avoiding potentially uncomfortable emotions by focusing on facts and logic. The situation is treated as an interesting problem that needs solving rationally, while the emotional complexities are

being ignored. We try to treat what feels emotionally unfathomable like an exam. For example, the recently redundant
worker creates endless spreadsheets and to-do lists, and attends
countless job interviews to avoid feelings of fear. The recent
singleton registers for every dating site, joins tennis, swimming
and pottery clubs and becomes busy with not feeling the feelings associated with loneliness. Infertility becomes a scientific
project to solve rather than sinking into the despair that might
be present.

Jargon is often used as a device to provide distance from
feelings. When we use complex terminology, the focus is on the
words, the concrete rather than the unfathomable emotional
landscape.

I (Jodie) worked with Amara (23) for 62 sessions. She
came to speak to me about her father's cancer diagnosis.
She wanted, it seemed, to tell me the story of her in-
depth research, her connection with experts and her
comprehensive knowledge of her dad's illness. I noticed
she was carrying a large bag with her to every session
and in our third session I asked her what was in it. She
took the contents out for me – the bag was filled with
reams of emails to experts, printouts of articles and books
on the body. She knew every single treatment, where to
get it, who the top surgeons were, and she would happily
recite this information to me and seem confident in doing
so. At first, it felt vital that I met her where she was and
supported the power she did have over the knowledge
she was finding, but after a number of sessions, I
interrupted her reading some text and said, 'You really

are amazing and you have so much knowledge, but this must be so hard for you. It really is upsetting what you're going through and you look so, so sad. It's OK to be sad here. Shall we maybe just stop for a minute?' At first, she was resistant to looking at me, looking more at the pages of her research, but when she was finally able to look up, she was so at sea in her feelings.

Over the weeks I suggested we portioned off the sessions, encouraging her to spend 60/40 on her week's findings and how she was feeling. Slowly we managed to use the majority of the sessions for her to connect with the parts of her that didn't have a clue what was happening, felt helpless, lost, sad and powerless; all of the things she could not connect with in her books and files. We were able to use her intellectualising her pain as a way into feeling. Had she not had the sessions, those feelings might well have emerged much later. I noticed over the weeks that her bag became smaller and smaller. She no longer carried around her grief, but had started to integrate it. Amara went on to begin her training with Macmillan Cancer Support.

Defence mechanisms are ultimately designed to support us. They allow us time and space before we become inundated by emotions and emotional content. However, if we don't create opportunities to get to know when we are using defence mechanisms and what forces are driving us to use them, if we don't create an environment where we are safe enough to come into contact with our feelings, push past and move through our defences, we remain unknown to ourselves.

We are unable to grow in the dark.
Self-knowledge shines lights.

How to Feel All the Feels

If we rely on defence mechanisms to help us survive emotionally, the pressure of our feelings amplifies, pushing against the defences until they become so powerful that they flood in regardless. Feelings will fight to be heard even in the most suppressing environments. What serves us better is finding ways to feel our feelings, so that they reduce in size rather than grow in energy. We all know that the monster under the bed only amplifies in fearsomeness the longer we don't look at it. The same can be applied to our feelings.

When we ignore our unconscious matter over prolonged periods of time, when we deny and ignore what feels too messy and uncomfortable, when we don't make space to process what's really going on for us, we shut ourselves off from our powerful regulating system. Ultimately we risk losing vital balance over our well-being. We do not give ourselves the opportunity to properly regulate and we disempower a system – the psyche – that is trying to keep us well. In doing so, we are mitigating data about ourselves that might be really useful to our consciousness and support our growth and well-being.

When we do not give ourselves space to think and feel deeply, we might begin to feel lethargic or overwhelmed at tasks we found manageable before; we might notice complexities in our relationships and feelings for others that are unrelenting and keep us away from intimacy. We might notice feeling more emotional, more irrational or much more sensitive or angry. We might find we misdirect frustrations. We might feel anxious, more depressed and/or experience a loss of joy over activities that once supported us to feel good. We might find our mental health suffers in various ways that might show up at first as stress or feelings of stress, but progress into much more paralysing mental health conditions over time. What serves us best is to take on the task of getting to know our unconscious and what it's trying to say.

'Until you make the unconscious conscious it'll direct
your life and you'll call it fate.' Jung

Things that make our emotions either get smaller or show up in ways that feel more manageable:

» embracing them
» getting curious about them
» owning them
» confronting them
» allowing them
» facing them
» naming/noting them
» being open to them
» honouring them

We may not be able to stop the hard feelings from showing up, but we can learn that we can tolerate what's hard. This allows them to move through us, rather than get stuck within us, residing underneath our many defence mechanisms. If we get to know our feelings, the range of our emotions, look out for their signs and traits, become friendlier, more familiar towards them, we'll be able to tend to them more effectively. So, how do you do that?

1. NOTICE WHAT'S HAPPENING IN YOUR BODY

Your body is such an intelligent instrument. However, when we are faced with difficult things, we can become disconnected from our bodies – some people describe this as 'out of body'. We don't notice what's happening in our bodies. Focusing on your physical self will really help ground you and bring you into the present.

Find ways of trying to describe what you're physically feeling. What does it feel like? For example:

» a pain in my chest
» a racing heart
» feeling hot and sweaty
» feeling confused
» a pit in my stomach
» palpitations/butterflies
» a headache
» feeling lost or confused
» feeling small
» looking for escapes (drink, drugs, sex, food)

2. TRY TO NAME IT

When we are having an intense emotional response, feeling at our limits, overwhelmed, anxious, nervous, disembodied or finding it hard to be present with ourselves, our limbic brain can start to pump stress hormones to our muscles to tighten and prepare us for action. This fight–flight mechanism is deeply wired inside our nervous system and takes over. This is a good thing to help protect ourselves if we are alone in a dark alley, but it's not a good thing if we are running a staff meeting and get angry at a co-worker.

Once you notice you are having a strong emotional reaction, or when you feel estranged or unsure about what you are feeling, the next step is to describe or name it – whether to yourself or out loud. For example, saying, 'I am feeling angry' or 'I have a tight ball of nerves in my gut.' Choosing words to describe subtle emotions jump-starts your executive brain and calms down your emotional limbic brain. From here, you can hover over your emotions, which gives your executive brain time to filter and organise your reactive, drama-filled emotions.

What names can you give to what you're feeling (try not to limit this to one – feelings rarely emerge in silo)? Call it what it is:

- » disappointment
- » guilt
- » sadness
- » anger
- » embarrassment
- » worry
- » pressure
- » fear
- » irritation
- » anxiety

3. NOTE TO SELF

Make some notes around what you experience in your body at times of adversity or even when you just feel a bit bleurgh. Sometimes, when we are in the heat of the moment, we can feel very different to times when we're more relaxed, so learning to identify that can help tell you what you need to do.

Things you might notice (though people have a huge variety):

»   'I feel hot and even standing at an open window doesn't help.'
»   'I'm drinking a lot, gulping water.'
»   'I feel clumsy, knocking things over.'
»   'I'm shuffling in my bag not sure what I'm looking for.'
»   'I can't remember people's names.'
»   'I need the loo loads.'
»   'I can't find things on my laptop, even though I know where they are.'
»   'I want to flick to social media.'
»   'I'm raising my voice.'
»   'My ears feel hot.'
»   'I'm coughing.'
»   'I'm saying things just for the sake of speaking.'
»   'I feel a bit out of control.'
»   'I want to eat something sugary.'

If you can voice some of these physical things, even to yourself, it helps connect you back to something tangible, so talk to yourself a little: 'Gosh my hands are sweaty, my heart's racing' and then reassure yourself that it's OK, it's going to pass.

Returning to a list you've made at times of feeling a lot can remind you that you have been here before, which reassures you that it will pass as it did before. Knowing or being more familiar with what's happening to you and in your body can ground you. It's affirming and helps you to be present.

4. TEND TO IT AS BEST YOU CAN

When children are distressed we are told the best way to make contact with them is to get down to their level, look them in the eye, hold their hands and reflect back to them what you see: 'You look really angry right now, this must be horrible for you, what do you need?' Can you do a version of this for yourself? Be your own best parent. Sit on the floor or as close to the floor as you can, or lean against a wall. Feel the support of what's there. Try to tune into that for a moment. Give yourself a hug. Look yourself in the eye, maybe in a mirror, or imagine it. Then try your best to name what you see. Then ask what would make you feel better right now, really better. For example, 'I just need to sit still/sleep/make that call/say that thing I need to say/ go outside for a minute/breathe.'

Allow the feeling a little space, time and attention. Don't rush too quickly to move past it by distracting yourself, but really allow yourself to sit with it. No one ever calmed down by being told to calm down, so do not expect that of yourself. Allow yourself to be a little at sea. Wrap yourself up in a blanket, drink water or a warm drink, lie on the floor, breathe deeply. Make space for the pictures in your mind to emerge, a little like daydreaming. What is emerging from your unconscious? Perhaps you can draw or write what you feel.

Don't punish yourself for being too sensitive or wallowing. Tending to feelings is a vital part of maintaining your mental health. Wallowing is submerging into something, and submerging into our feelings can be deeply cathartic and beneficial.

5. BE REALISTIC

Don't expect miracles and magic Tipp-Ex pens for your complexities. We are all learning. It is OK at times just to know you are feeling something. You don't have to be too prescriptive about your outcomes. Say out loud: 'I'm feeling something right now and it's difficult' or 'I don't feel good right now.' Sometimes voicing what's going on for yourself is enough to give you permission to feel deeper.

6. BE A TOURIST

When encouraging yourself to feel, don't treat it like a test to be completed. Instead, allow yourself the opportunity to amble around, tripping, exploring, making the wrong turns. Think of yourself as a tourist to your emotions. Stop often for rest and refreshments, light and shade, enjoy the sun and trinkets. Holiday a little away from the harsh realities of having to have it all together. Allow yourself the luxury of mess (do you find your holiday room is much less organised than your house?), sand on your feet, damp swimwear, tingly skin. Allow yourself the possibility of discovering something new, however daunting.

We aren't perfect, infallible robots. In the same way we know that eating pizza three nights in a row is going to make us feel like crap, sometimes we do it anyway. In the same way we know deep down that not saying what we need can make us feel physically unwell, distracted, upset and alone, sometimes we still do it. Sometimes we do not feel worth the effort, we do not feel good enough; sometimes we are exhausted from constantly doing the work. We cannot treat ourselves as never-ending self-improvement projects – sometimes we need a rest from ourselves. Sometimes we need to repeat habits that make us feel worse in order to remember how bad that feels. Sometimes we sabotage our own progress in order to remember the safety of the old, even if it is uncomfortable and destructive. Sometimes we get into relationships with people who aren't good for us, sometimes we drink too much. Sometimes we shout at our kids, and sometimes we send a shitty email to our boss. We don't sleep enough, we overcommit, we overspend, we get in a mess. And that's OK!

Feeling our feelings is really hard and sometimes we just can't bear it. We will do anything to avoid it. As we've explored, this might manifest in lifelong defence and coping mechanisms. Our job, then, is to keep enquiring about what is really serving us and question habits and behaviours that really aren't in order to change them. Change and our ability to make changes is what keeps us flexible. When we are rigid we become brittle, breakable, but when we are softer, we are stronger.

Chapter 4

Childhood Matters

There is no such thing as an uneventful childhood. Each of us has our own personal history, which is made up of strong events or experiences that impact us dramatically, and also subtle looks or sentences that are uttered by our parents or caregivers. Many of us hold a belief that our childhoods were relatively uneventful and that nothing 'big' or out of the ordinary happened. Because of this, we often have a hard time understanding our behaviour. Talking about our childhood in therapy may seem clichéd – 'Tell me about your parents' we've seen in many memes – but really this is where our core belief system has its foundations. By giving time and attention to unpacking what has gone before for us, where we have come from and who we are – as uninspiring, happy or horrible as we might remember it – we can collect really useful data about ourselves. We all have the opportunity to learn about ourselves if we want to and can face it. In learning we might be able to encourage ourselves to shed some unhelpful thoughts, ideas and feelings we harbour from our childhoods that are keeping us stuck. We might be able to get respite from behaviours that aren't helping us grow, or reach out to our younger selves with the compassion we've been needing to help us feel a bit better. When we understand some of the factors that contribute to who we are today, we colour ourselves in a little more, we become and feel more 3D, we fill out. We are then able to use the sustenance to grow through what we've been through.

Most people don't want their childhoods to matter but, invariably, they do. Each of us has a rich, personal history that begins as early as in the womb. This is made up of dramatic events or experiences that may hit us like a ton of bricks, and also more subtle moments that have the ability to linger and stay with us across our entire lifetime.

Let's Talk About Trauma

After meeting thousands of people within our work, we have come to the conclusion that there is no such thing as an uneventful childhood; no such thing as an upbringing without at least one wounding experience.

'ACE' is an acronym that would be familiar to most qualified therapists. It came out of a large public health study – the Adverse Childhood Experiences Study – conducted in the mid nineties by the Center for Disease Control and the Kaiser Permanente healthcare organisation in California.

The study measured ten types of childhood trauma. Some were personal: physical abuse, verbal abuse, sexual abuse, physical neglect and emotional neglect. Some were related to parents, caregivers or other family members: a family member who's an alcoholic, a victim of domestic violence, in prison, diagnosed with a mental illness or going through a divorce. Each type of trauma counts as one. So, if you're a person whose parent/caregiver had depression, if you were verbally abused and your parents divorced before you were 18, you would have an ACE score of 3.

About 17,000 people took part in the ACE study and the researchers found, firstly, that two-thirds of them had at least one adverse childhood experience and secondly, that whatever happened to them in their childhood would have a physical, social, emotional or health impact later in life. In other words, what happened to them would stay with them in some way.

'Subtle' trauma

When we think about difficult childhoods, our minds race to the traumas measured in this ACE study – stories of children who are beaten, sexually abused, screamed at, blamed or humiliated. We're so used to focusing on the horrors of abuse that come from intentional, physical and abrupt action, that we forget about those equally painful moments of inaction: of neglect or ignoring.

On the surface, everything may have appeared fine, but hidden underneath other provisions of care and necessities like a roof over your head, material things or a routine, the adverse childhood experiences you might have had might have been subtle and unmemorable. A parent or caregiver may not have been very affectionate and cuddles or moments of embrace may have been few and far between. They may not have shown much interest in you, how your day was at school, why you came home looking sad. They may have always had something more urgent to do: work to get on with or a place to be. They may not have lifted their heads to look at you when reading the paper. They may not have held your gaze. In an effort to be 'perfect parents', they may have modelled constant excelling and overachieving as a standard and bar to reach, leaving you little room to be real, and feeling like a failure for not meeting those standards. They may have left you for another family at a very early stage in your life. They may have been totally shut off from their own emotions or been unable to regulate them. They may have told you (directly or indirectly) that you can't or shouldn't experience certain emotions. When you got angry or upset, you may have been given a time out and left isolated on the 'naughty step', forced to contend with your need to be close and attached to them and your need to authentically feel and express your emotions.

Whatever it was for you, any of the above or something else, however obvious or subtle the challenges of your childhood were, they hold validity and are worth giving time to be thought and felt about. They stay with you, even if your parents did do their best. The trauma isn't necessarily the thing that happens, or in the cases of inaction, doesn't happen, but it is what happens inside of you as a result of these traumatic events. The trauma is that you become disconnected from your emotions, intuition and from your body. The trauma is having difficulty being in the present moment. It is developing a negative view of your body and a negative view of the world. It is not knowing what you need, like or want. It is losing your sense of self. It is developing a defensive view of people. It is people-pleasing in order to feel seen. It is drinking or doing drugs to regulate emotions that went unregulated and unsupported. It is mistrusting others, pushing them away, avoiding close relationships. It is being terrified of rejection and uncomfortable showing affection.

The more time we spend denying or avoiding the reality of these experiences, the more of a hard time we have understanding our behaviour. We experience so much shame for the dysfunctional and destructive patterns we find ourselves acting out in adulthood because we had, on the whole, 'supportive families'. We experience this shame, confusion and misunderstanding because the challenges of our childhood are broader, more nuanced and more complex than we account for.

The more we can look at our childhoods with care, compassion and curiosity, the less likely we are to unconsciously rely on maladaptive patterns or ways of coping when we face challenges in adult life. The more we can get in touch with our sensations and the feelings in our body (our breath, the tension we carry, any heat we feel), the more we can get in touch with and release what we carry with us from our pasts. From here, we can take more control. From here, we can lessen the negative impact our childhoods have on our adult relationships, especially our relationship with our own children, our intimate partners and ourselves. (If you feel you need more support, please see the list of resources on page 320.)

POSITIVE EXPERIENCES IN CHILDHOOD

As important as it is to have a sensitivity towards ACEs, it's equally important to hold an awareness of PACEs too. Developed by Jennifer Hays-Grudo and Amanda Sheffield Morris, PACEs are 'Protective and Compensatory Experiences' that can boost our resilience and mitigate the risks that come with ACEs. They can be broken down into two main categories: relationships and resources.

Relationships:
» feeling safe and secure in attachments
» receiving unconditional love
» opportunities to connect socially with others
» feeling a sense of belonging to
» having other adults to look up to
» having caregivers who can help you understand, regulate and validate your emotions

Resources:
» having a good and predictable routine
» access to education and a support network
» living in a clean, safe home with enough food
» doing sports or exercise
» volunteering in the community or contributing to something positively

JOURNAL PROMPT

What positive childhood experiences did you have? How much or how often during your childhood did you:

» feel able to talk to your family about feelings?
» feel your family stood by you during difficult times?
» enjoy participating in community traditions?
» feel a sense of belonging in school?
» feel supported by friends?

» have at least two non-parent adults who took a genuine interest in you?

» feel safe and protected by an adult in your home?

The Impact of Emotional Neglect

Experiencing emotional messiness or disorder as children – confusing, shaming, upsetting things that were not tended to or just things that didn't make sense – without some thought or care extended towards them, can remain just that – a mess.

Whatever it was for you, however subtle, having our emotions going under-noticed, undervalued or under-responded to stays with us and lingers across our lifetime. Invariably and unavoidably, it has a lasting impact. We experience a few things as a result of this:

WE BECOME DISCONNECTED FROM OUR EMOTIONS

The powerful, energising feedback system which should be stimulating, directing, guiding, informing, connecting and enriching us – our emotions, which should be telling us who matters to us and what matters to us, and why – becomes disconnected. Our emotions become less like bright signals showing us the way, and become fainter and flickering, sending out broken Morse code. It is here that we might begin to feel stuck – stuck in situations that we don't really want to be in; trapped in far from good-enough relationships; living situations that aren't ideal; jobs in which we feel overlooked and undervalued; friendships that don't serve us . . . the list goes on.

WE HIDE FROM OUR EMOTIONS (AND HIDE OURSELVES)

'It is a joy to be hidden, but a disaster not to be found.' Donald Winnicott

We regularly think of this quote when we come across people who are well hidden or defended, from themselves and from the rest of the world (and at the same time, are really sad about it). Hiding is a strategy that we deploy to take care of ourselves. We learn that emotions aren't safe. We learn that crying is not appreciated. We learn that life runs more smoothly when we pack our emotions into our ribcage and forget about them. We learn that it's best not to take up too much space, that it's best to hide away. Yet, similar to children playing hide-and-seek, we long to be found, to be seen, to be heard and to be validated. This is the same for infants, children and adults alike. There is nothing worse than hearing the game going on around you and feeling that nobody cares enough to come and find you. We all seek relationships with others where we feel that we are recognised and valued for being ourselves. However, for those of us who have not been recognised as children or feel we have never been seen or truly recognised, it can be both a terrifying and alluring possibility.

OUR HIDDEN EMOTIONS REMAIN UNADDRESSED AND UNMANAGED

To cope as a child, we push our emotions down to keep them from becoming a 'problem' for our parents. We learn that we must wall off our own emotions so that we will never appear sad, hurt, needy or emotional. Those blocked emotions just sit there, unattended to, waiting, perhaps emerging at times which seem to make little sense to us. Or maybe they don't emerge at all, but instead, negatively impact our relationships or choices.

OUR BODIES ARE IMPACTED

We know that 'what we resist persists'. The more something is ignored, the more it will fight for attention. When feelings and emotions are ignored, they amplify and get stronger. They also find surprising, abrupt and potentially destructive ways of emerging, such as physical or verbal aggression, crying over seemingly unimportant things, losing our temper quickly, falling in 'love' often, becoming obsessed with others, past or future events and/ or developing a disproportionate connection to world events.

But they also manifest internally as psychological incongruence. This is when someone feels and expresses their inner emotions in an inconsistent manner with their outer world – through their speech and body language. As an example, have you ever smiled when you're talking about something sad? Or felt very emotional, yet had a flat face and still posture? Have you ever felt angry, but pushed it down and developed a headache? These are incongruent speech and behaviour patterns.

Incongruence happens when we've lost touch with our inner world and our emotions are represented with bodily sensations. Emotions are unavoidable and they will find a way of being heard if we don't give them the attention they need.

I (Jodie) worked with Deepak (27) for 34 sessions. He came to see me because he said he felt embarrassed that he cried so easily. He said it felt like it was involuntary

and he was triggered often. He was particularly
concerned that he could not watch a film with even
the slightest theme of upset in. Because he became so
distressed, there was hardly anything outside of some
Disney films he could tolerate. He had a physical response
to being in a cinema or seeing content in a magazine
that was at all upsetting. He would get dizzy, feel faint
and need to lie down.

I noticed in our sessions that it was rare for him to
associate or share feelings of upset or distress in his
everyday life and he often spoke about this being fine
and life feeling fairly easy (apart from this trouble). I
began to wonder if perhaps he was disassociating from
what felt hard and upsetting in his life, brushing it off and
disallowing his feelings, meaning his emotions needed a
vehicle for space and attention and they had locked on
to something that felt relevant, like provocative material,
to find a way into the light. With this in mind, I began to
encourage him to engage more with the reality of his life,
the nuances, so that he could start to articulate and feel
feelings as they emerged.

During our work together, as things started to integrate
more for him with feelings emerging where we might
expect them (an argument with his boyfriend, a failed job
application, conflict with his brother), he was able to tell me
that when he was 11 his best friend who lived two doors up
had been hit by a bus and died. He had not been able to
process his complex and overwhelming feelings about this
at the time, but had instead reverted to watching endless
movies to drown out his sorrow. Most likely his body had

stored his grief and his psyche was in some way processing it, tears were falling and he felt upset, but he located this as being connected to other people's stories (films). In turn, this gave him some control over his big emotions: 'I won't watch a film as I don't want to feel sad.' We kept working on his everyday associations and feelings and soon he was feeling a range of emotions across his life and his physical film triggers became more proportionate.

The body does keep the score: you may notice at times of high emotion that you have a tummy ache or headaches. Or when life is feeling hard you might bang your head or twist an ankle, finding a way of somehow halting you, drawing attention to the pain.

OUR RELATIONSHIPS ARE IMPACTED

We might come to mistrust ourselves and believe that all of the answers can be found within another. We believe that we're not good enough. We shame ourselves for feeling and deny our own experiences. We cut off, disassociate, distract and pacify ourselves. We unconsciously seek out romantic relationships that recreate the conflicted dynamic we had with our parents. We find ourselves in behaviour patterns that are familiar yet uncomfortable yet we feel unable to make change (see page 27 for more on this).

Our Core Beliefs

Much of what we are in contact with as adults has its foundations in our early experiences. We formulate core beliefs that, unchallenged, can stay with us for life. Perhaps you grew up in a household that didn't celebrate diversity, that disregarded learning or that disrespected authority or rules. What kind of impact does that have on the way you live now? We inherit core beliefs, regardless of how useful they are to our growth, progress or sense of thriving.

Core beliefs are our most deeply held assumptions about ourselves, others and the world. They are born from our early experiences and are most often passed on through our systemic or family beliefs. They are deeply embedded in our thinking and significantly shape our perception of the world and our way of being. They often go unnoticed yet constantly influence our lives.

Core beliefs can be the root cause of many of our difficulties, including negative thinking and poor decision-making. Yet, as the name suggests, core beliefs are exactly that – beliefs rather than facts (though often we believe they are facts). They may be untrue, no longer relevant or do very little to serve us. They can also be self-fulfilling prophesies, particularly if they live deeply in our unconscious. For example, if we grew up in an environment where others were viewed as threatening to our safety and we internalised the belief that 'people are generally untrustworthy and do not want the best for me', it is possible that we will look for this in the world and attract people who affirm our belief. Children who move around a lot, country to country or school to school, might internalise the belief that places aren't for staying in, that it's boring to stay in one place for too long or that relationships are transitional. They might, as adults, move often, even though it's exhausting and they crave commitment, because this is what they have always done, this is how they know how to be in the world. They justify their decisions by convincing themselves it feels good (and maybe it does some of the time).

> I (Jodie) worked with Alina (52) for over 60 sessions. Alina came to see me because she felt that sex and intimacy with her partner of 12 years was strained and inhibited and she wanted to feel more confident and liberated in this area of her relationship. In her own words, she felt she was 'fearful of her own pleasure' and this was negatively impacting her life. She grew up in a Christian family and was the middle of seven siblings. She quickly and readily shared early on in our work – something we later identified as at the centre of her complex – that when she was in her teens, her mother suffered significant illness caused by pain in the abdomen and had a hysterectomy with complications. Alina reflects on this time as being shrouded in shame somehow and that there was a sense in the household of her mother's illness being somehow dirty. Things were not openly discussed and during this time Alina was not allowed access to her mum. She remembers it as a chaotic time too where she had lots of caring duties for her siblings and she felt her family was struggling to keep going without her mother's care. She felt isolated and alone.
>
> We spent some weeks compassionately reflecting how this was for her. She was able to make some emotional sense of an upbringing that had little liberation around sex or sexuality within it due to religious beliefs and family values, where devout beliefs were upheld. It was

suggested, though not explicitly said, that the illness was related to the fact that her mother was not a virgin at the time of marriage and there was a suggestion she was being punished for this. This had significantly impacted Alina's relationship with her body, her libido and her thoughts and feelings around sex.

Alina's inherited core beliefs, although she did not align with these consciously as an adult (she did not live as a Christian or practise faith), had a significant impact on her mental health and her life in the present. We were able to realign her thoughts and relationship to her pleasure and liberated her away from some of her unhelpful core beliefs. It's important to say here, though, that this work was persistent for her and it took much work every day to maintain some growth.

Our core beliefs often seem at first as if they serve us very well. We feel familiar and secure in holding them. They ground us to something. They give us a place to orientate ourselves from, either passionately accepting our belief systems or acting out against them. But, in many cases, core beliefs are unhelpful and at odds with a real sense of contentedness. We might feel reassured by the familiarity of what we find ourselves in, yet also hold a belief that we are not reaching our own potential or are journeying down paths not meant for us. We can convince ourselves that it's much more productive for us to continue with what we know than to challenge or change it. We can convince ourselves that we are 'happy' where we're at, so that we don't have to face a realm unknown to us – something different.

Keeping your core beliefs unexplored and leaving them unchallenged can, in some cases, contribute to poor mental health. Mental maintenance (see page 19) will help you to grow and use your experiences to better navigate the future. We are going to look now at how core beliefs can manifest, and share some ways you can begin to overcome them to encourage yourself into growth.

LIMITING SELF-BELIEFS

When our core beliefs limit us, it can be difficult to spot exactly what's happening. For example, we might notice that we find growth incredibly hard or change near-on impossible. It's useful to think about how this is showing up in your life so that it's possible to get underneath it.

If one of my core beliefs suggests that the world is a dangerous place, my coping mechanism might look like agoraphobia at one end of the scale or an inability to do anything other than go to work and back home again. A core belief might very well inform the way we understand, accept or disassociate from our feelings. If, within your family, being emotional was frowned upon or laughed at or if nobody modelled talking about how they felt, it might give you a false belief that you aren't able to or are underequipped to manage complex emotional situations, having never been given the opportunity to try. For example, many children are overprotected from death, excluded from the detail that might be helpful to them in later life. They become fearful of what was perceived as fearful on their behalf.

TIME FOR REFLECTION

» Were you overprotected from divorce, death, house moves, job loss or other difficult life situations as a child?

» How has that left you feeling now?

Our core belief systems can motivate us towards unusual habits and behaviours. Perhaps we were told we were stupid, naughty, loud, incompetent, untrustworthy, boring, frumpy, clumsy or stinky. Perhaps we understand this as 'fact' and therefore we welcome in and fulfil our beliefs – we misbehave, overeat, don't speak out at parties, because somewhere deeply we believe what we have been told.

One client, who found it very difficult to create healthy habits for herself, shared that, 'My father won't walk in the park with me, because he thinks that if we start walking and talking I might cry and he doesn't want people to see me crying.' Here we have a very unhelpful set of core values passed on generationally. One which says firstly, 'I choose others' views over your well-being', secondly, that crying is somehow thought of as negative and shameful, and thirdly, a push for repression of feelings. What he is also saying is – if you want time with me, you need to be a certain way; I don't accept your mess. We might wonder here about the father's own core beliefs, which might consider crying as weak, and that confidence is built on what others think of him.

We also see unhelpful core beliefs in relationship difficulties. If you grew up in a family that believed in 'traditional' marriage, heterosexuality or women as sole caregivers, then challenging these core values can cause massive emotional upset for individuals. It's something we see in the therapy room frequently – unhappiness in relationships being untended because the idea of coming into contact with an imperfect marriage, even for yourself, is too unbearable. We become bound up in a set of values that do not liberate us into feeling, into change, into growth, but keep us paralysed in beliefs we might not even understand why we hold on to.

DO YOU FEEL 'GOOD ENOUGH'?

A common core belief that people arrive at therapy with is feeling 'not good enough, flawed, disappointing, unworthy' and a whole host of negative assumptions and beliefs that have nothing to do with how they actually are in the world. They can experience feelings of not being good enough as a wife, parent, employee, boss, friend, child . . . the list goes on.

You might have a gnawing feeling that hangs around you that you don't feel good enough. Perhaps you measure your feeling of being good enough against your output or on what others say, but perhaps even when your output is good or you hear positive things you don't feel any more enough? There isn't any hard evidence that you are not enough, but still you feel it. So where do your feelings of not being good enough come from?

If you grew up in a household where people didn't feel good enough, where you heard or sensed very low confidence, where a low sense of self-worth or esteem was evident, manifest perhaps in your caregivers, it will have oriented your belief systems towards a sense of not being good enough. If it was directed at or projected on to you, it might be even more evident in your day today. Perhaps you were told you weren't good enough or were disappointing by a caregiver. Or you couldn't fix a challenging situation at home and you internalised a sense of this being your fault, that you were not good enough to fix it or make it better (this can be particularly true for the child of addicts or where domestic violence was present).

Caregivers may have been struggling with their own feelings, unable to articulate how they were feeling about their parenting role or life stage – helpless, useless, inadequate, angry and not good enough feelings might all have been sent into the shadow parts of themselves, too frightening to be integrated. These might then have emerged as projections on to you as a child or young adult, which can give you feelings of inadequacy, fear, anger and anxiety which don't truthfully belong to you.

Your very early life will have had an impact on how you feel about yourself. Postnatal and postpartum depression is, only in recent years, something that has been tended to with care and empathy. Those who struggled to bond with their children were often left alone with their negative and upsetting thoughts, which may well be projected on to the baby/child. You have feelings as an adult of not being good enough, yet you can't quite trace the source or identify how you are not good enough – there is a lack of evidence. This might suggest this has been inherited unconsciously from early years; disowning it or reframing it will take some work through everyday mental maintenance (see page 19).

We all have experience of feeling not good enough at times. This is part of being human. But really trying to understand *why* you don't feel good enough can be really helpful in understanding what might be contributing to your growth being hindered.

What Are Your Core Beliefs?

Understanding yourself, who you really are, gives you a deep sense of confidence. It prepares you to fully accept what you like about yourself and to know what's serving you, and what isn't. Understanding your own core beliefs is an essential way in which you can grow from where you've been and take ownership over who you are becoming.

TIME FOR REFLECTION

Take some time to sit with a notebook and ask yourself the questions below. By all means, write the first answer that comes into your head, but go on and challenge yourself to think a little deeper. You are not trying to impress anyone here, so take a deeper dive into the flowing water with all the possibilities that might be there:

» How do I view myself, in three words?
» What does my inner voice sound like/say often?
» How do I feel when good things happen in my life?
» How do I feel when bad things happen in my life?
» How do I mostly view myself:
    > at work?
    > as a partner/friend?
    > as a parent/sibling/son/daughter?
» How do I feel mostly about others and their achievements?

» Do I categorise people in the world? If so, how?

Notice how you answer. Which of those came easily and which less so? What do you feel about what you see?

Now challenge what you've just uncovered. Have a look at the list you have made and see what factual evidence you have that these are true.

» Create a column that evidences your statements and list all of the things that cement what you believe about yourself.
» Ask someone you trust (a therapist, partner, friend or colleague) to comment on your statements (don't ask someone who has been part of your belief-forming). Discuss what they've written and enquire about their experience of you.
» Review your list of core beliefs and ask, 'Is this some-thing my caregiver also believes/says?'
» Now create a list of everything that disputes your statement. List the factual evidence in your life.
» Notice if your beliefs about yourself and the world change if you are more stressed, facing life changes or anxious about something. Notice what's happening in your life and how that impacts your beliefs.

Is what you have found surprising, uncomfortable or familiar? Know that however hard it feels, knowledge is the power in the tank that will fuel your growth.

HOW TO CHANGE YOUR NEGATIVE CORE BELIEFS

What you are asking of yourself is a reorientation away from what you've known and what's kept you safe (but perhaps limited) for many years. Don't expect it to happen easily. In the same way caged animals set free often find it difficult to leave the cage to explore the wild, you need to treat your new landscape, and feelings towards it, with caution, empathy, love and tenderness. Know that it'll feel uncomfortable. It might even feel like loss, not gain, at first. You might feel confused, uncertain and disbelieving in the process. Know that you may well come up against some very uncomfortable feelings about people you love and that conflict might emerge as you begin to change. Know that there is nothing quick and easy about change. But it is worth it. We grow through change; just like growing pains as teenagers, changing is also energising and hopeful. It gives you a new understanding of yourself and the people in your world. It will ultimately bring you closer to yourself.

Know that your own change and growth can be really destabilising for the people closest to you – family, friends, acquaintances, even colleagues; they can feel left out, frightened, terrified of their own stuckness, resentful of your growth, jealous of your change, and they might revert to reminding you of the old core values, such as, 'This is so you, to not care about anyone else but yourself' or 'Here we go again with all your therapy talk' or 'You'll be bored of this soon like you always are.'

How, then, can you stay committed to your change? How can you find space to listen to what is being said or what has perhaps frequently been said and let it go? Changing any negative and unhelpful core belief involves adapting a long-held, often

emotionally laden, point of view, which has been a fundamental part of your identity for many years. Know that you'll have
setbacks and fall into old habits. Know that it's OK to test things
out, fail and try again.

Create compassionate alternatives
When a negative core belief is mobilised it can be incredibly
powerful and difficult to interrupt. You will find numerous ways
to support your own failures or give more energy to the core
belief that you are wedded to (even unwillingly). You might find
that you can interpret almost anything to support the unhelpful
belief. Compassionate alternatives can help counter this.

> I (Jodie) saw Zehra (30) over 12 sessions, who had a
> negative view of the way she looked. I asked her to write
> down comments that others had said about her, during
> the week, that disproved her belief. She collected 17
> comments such as, 'You look lovely', 'That colour really
> suits you', 'Where did you get that dress? I love it' and so
> on. Shortly after sharing the list, she went on to reassure
> herself that people were 'Only saying that because they
> felt they had to'. So now we had two core beliefs! The
> second one being that 'People only say what they think
> you want to hear'.
>
> We could now begin to move away from Zehra
> identifying with validation that was around how she
> looked – this was a core belief from her upbringing,
> around the way women needed to look. We then looked
> at how she felt about others, how others made her feel
> and what impact she had on them. We were able to move

closer to real meaning for her in the world and past a core belief that was keeping her in a more superficial and lonely space.

TIME FOR REFLECTION

Ask yourself:

» What am I telling myself right now?
» Is this helping me or hindering me?
» What would be the opposite of getting in the way of myself? (For example, bigging myself up or loving myself.)
» How might that sound? ('I am doing my best and what I need is X to support me.')

Can you keep reiterating and repeating this exercise to challenge your core belief out of its power? This might feel really absurd at the start and you might feel resistant to even trying. Try to push through and keep at it even when it feels ridiculous.

Talk about what you're doing

It can be really helpful to create some allies who you can share the journey with. These might be friends, a trusted family member, a therapist or even a work colleague who you align with. Share with them what you've noticed about yourself and how you are hoping to change. You might choose to share your past, how the core belief was created through your lived experience. Share some ideas about how you want to make it different. Ask for support. This is a lovely way to create intimacy and make good relationships great.

This might sound like:

» 'My relationship with food is really tricky. I have an idea that I don't deserve things that are good for me. I'm trying to change that, so can you keep an eye on what I'm picking up at lunch and suggest alternatives?'

» 'I was often told that my opinion doesn't matter. I know I want to have more confidence in my voice. If I put myself down or go quiet can you flick me on the arm?'

» 'I was told men were a threat and predatory when I was younger. I'm hoping to get more confidence around my relationship with men. Can you support me with that by inviting me into conversations with men?'

Give yourself time and space

Core beliefs are often learnt and then enmeshed, galvanised and cemented over years, so don't expect these to alter easily. Once you let a dog on the sofa, it's almost impossible to keep it off. Treat yourself how you would that dog – keep encouraging yourself away from what isn't useful, or what you don't want, and invite yourself into something new. Give yourself time and space to unpick and be curious about your beliefs – the helpful and the unhelpful. Question, probe and tease out what makes you *you*. Even just being curious and identifying your core beliefs is a massive step towards evolution.

*

It can be so empowering to identify these early influences on your thought processes, self-esteem and core beliefs. Once you recognise something about yourself, you can begin to apply yourself towards doing it differently.

PART 2

Mental Maintenance in Practice

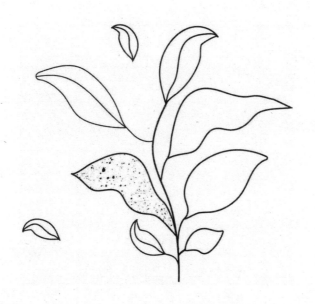

These next pages are an invitation to practise some of our suggestions for mental maintenance – the every day, every week practices that will support your growth in the right direction. We believe that with mental maintenance grows a confidence in your ability to get through challenges, knowing that while things might not be perfect, your work is paying off.

Better mental health is a practice, not a destination.

As toddlers we spend an enormous amount of time wobbling around and falling over until we find our feet. It's how we get to know what sharp edges to avoid, how we find our balance through our imbalance. It is the same with our mental well-being. We understand feeling better from our experiences of feeling worse. As we did with our first steps, our task here is to practise at our better mental health, knowing that it isn't a linear journey towards success and that success is not the big gold medal at the end. Instead, let's celebrate smaller personal triumphs and gently tend to falls.

Much of our mental health is responsive to our environment, our relationships and what's happening in our lives. Creating the right environment to be your most conscious and engaged self takes practice on a regular basis. Just like yoga, riding or swimming, the less we practice, the less good we'll be, and the less strength and stamina we'll have. Sometimes it will feel good, sometimes it will feel tricky or boring. Sometimes it will feel hopeless and you'll abandon your commitment to yourself. But each time you *commit to practice*, you commit to opening up the opportunity for growth. Each time you return you show self-compassion: that you matter, that you are worth it.

We are acutely aware that sometimes when we are faced with a 'to-do' list of tasks it can feel awful, like unwanted homework, a complete overload to the system. Have a little moment to ask what time you have available to yourself for your mental maintenance – a minute, an hour, a day, a week, a year, ongoing? And honour your capacity.

We will not always get our self-care right. Try not to sabotage the progress you may have made by beating yourself up if you don't get it right all of the time. Knocking your own confidence in the way you speak to and think about yourself depletes the precious resources you need for your own growth.

> Sometimes we will not practise behaviour
> that supports our better mental health . . .
> Because we are human!

We have identified four areas for mental maintenance practice, and we will have a chapter on each of them in this part of the book:

1. The foundations
2. Proper self-care

3. Routine and rituals

4. Replenish

There are no quick fixes with mental maintenance, but you *can* aim for longer periods of contentment in your life. You *can* find more moments of joy, connectedness and meaning. You *can* reach a greater sense of confidence in your true self, along with more consciousness about what you are doing, feeling and saying, and why. In building this self-understanding, we hope that you feel better equipped to manage life's adversities, and when you do feel horrible, alone and struggling (which we all do, at times), you can be more sure of what you need to do to help yourself feel better.

Chapter 5

The Foundations

Here is the shit you will undoubtedly know already, but we are going to say it anyway, mostly because we'd be negligent not to. Every single time a person sits in one of our therapy chairs feeling their lowest, their most out of control, their saddest, most hopeless, every single time we ourselves are lying awake anxious or overwhelmed, if we ask the basic questions: 'Did you drink water today?', 'Are you sleeping?', 'Have you stretched?', 'Have you breathed fresh air?', 'Have you rested?' the answer is almost always a resounding 'no'.

The foundations to good mental maintenance are the least sexy thing ever, but without them we are tumbleweed, floating along unanchored, tripping over our belief that we are unable to feel better. **We know this stuff contributes to better mental health.** So keep reminding yourself that you need to do these things, even when you feel at your worst. In fact, it's a priority when you feel at your worst – these things are necessary acts of self-love. They are micro-communications to yourself that you matter. They often don't fill us with immediate joy and can feel a bit like cleaning the oven – boring as hell and unappealing – but we know we'll feel better after.

Check In With Yourself

Let's start with a morning check-in. The following exercise has been inspired by one in the brilliant *Conscious Uncoupling* by Katherine Woodward Thomas. Take five minutes to really notice where you're at.

» Sit on the bed, on the floor or against a wall. Close your eyes for a minute and relax your shoulders, your forehead your jaw and notice your breath.

» Count your breaths in for three and out for three until you feel yourself settle down.

» You might want to position yourself in front of the mirror so that you can see yourself. Ask yourself, even speak the words aloud: 'How do you feel my love?' You might find it difficult to speak to yourself in this way, with a sense of real care and affection. Notice if using endearing terms like 'my love' or 'darling' to speak to yourself feels uncomfortable, cheesy even; wonder about that, or find a term that you feel is nurturing to you.

» Allow your feelings to emerge. The list might be quite long, but give them a voice and name them one by one: 'I feel jealous, lost, angry, unsure . . . I don't know.'

» Allow those to sink in, then ask yourself, 'What do you need my love?'

» Allow yourself to answer: 'I need rest, food, validation, to say something unsaid, to breath more.' Sometimes it doesn't come easily and you'll want to jump up and move away or avoid it. Try to stay with it and let what is there emerge.

» Try to find a closing affirmation that speaks to you. It might sound like: 'You deserve all of that and more.' 'I am enough.' 'I am feeling but I am not my feelings.' 'Feelings come and go, they are transient, but I am here.'

This practice is really helpful in getting us closer to ourselves. It gives voice to what is inside and sets the tone for our self-worth: 'What I feel and need matters, and is worth listening to.'

Sleep

It is night-time, but sleep won't come. You turn over. You turn the pillow over, the cold side. One leg out of the bed, one leg in. Perhaps a different position will turn down the volume on the overthinking. Frustration sets in. Tomorrow's tasks flash before your eyes. You play back your day. You play back an argument you had ages ago. You win it this time. You begin to existentially ponder the big stuff: What am I doing? Where am I going?

Not being able to sleep is hell. Many of us share in this. We asked over 2,000 in the Self Space community about their sleeping habits:

» 87 per cent still felt tired when they woke up in the morning.
» 64 per cent had regular awakenings during the night.
» 55 per cent struggled to get to sleep at night.
» 59 per cent were bothered by waking up too early and not being able to get back to sleep.

Sleep is so important. A night of restful sleep has a restorative function, that optimises our creative and cognitive performance for the next day. It equips us to be better able to handle emotional challenges, too. Sleep really does contribute to our better mental health; it balances out our consciousness and makes difficult things feel possible. Try to keep sleep as a powerful, and the most available, gift you can give yourself.

Sleep is the place where your consciousness restores balance through your unconscious mind. Often if things are unattended to in your conscious life they'll emerge in your unconscious. Treat your sleeplessness in some cases as communication that some things need looking at, tending to and enquiring about (see also later our thoughts on dreams – page 145).

Our culture doesn't 'reward' us for good sleep. Instead, busyness is worn as a badge of honour. We skip lunch, work

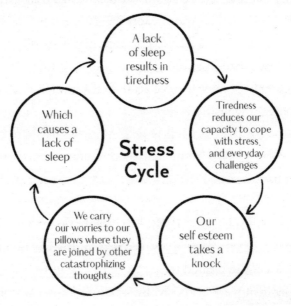

The sleep–stress cycle

late, check our phones . . . But on our hamster wheels of over-commitment, we forget that inside our weary adult bodies exists an inner child that needs and deserves to sleep. Even when it feels like it doesn't want to. It doesn't have to always be this way. Whether you're reading this in the harsh light of day or in the lonely dead of night, we can search together for a balm for those nocturnal niggles. Maybe you're trying to navigate a small baby, a demanding toddler or a noisy neighbour. Maybe you are a carer and hypervigilance is something you feel you need. Perhaps you're up against a tough deadline or working night shifts or managing shifting sleep patterns for work outside your time zone. How do you stay well when sleep is what you know you need, but life does not allow it?

» **Share the load:** Can you find a way for the sleeplessness not to be endless and continuous? This could look like splitting shifts, having a rota with a co-parent or sibling, or staying away at a friend's house. Can you build in times where you know you will be able to sleep?
» **Lower the expectations of yourself:** At times when sleep is limited, set your diary to 'less busy' and don't pile on more tasks.
» **Allow others in:** Being overtired is something almost all of us can relate to. Be honest with others about your real-ity and how at your limits you are feeling, so that you can manage the expectations of those around you.
» **Rest when you can:** Even if sleep is not possible, sit for longer and give your mind and body an opportunity to settle.
» **Prioritise yourself:** Really notice when you are putting the needs of others above your own. Work out what behaviour

is people-pleasing and doing you a disservice (making you feel like shit) and what is unavoidable. We can't leave a baby unattended, but we can call and ask a friend to watch them for an hour, or leave the washing so we can sleep when they do. Know when you are sleep-deprived and try to give yourself a little of what you need.

SLEEP LIKE A BABY

Take a moment to reflect on how much care and attention parents of young children put into their child's sleep routines. It is a sweet science and an art. The blackout blinds, the white noise machine, the monitoring of the room temperature, plenty of naps during the day and early nights are a must. They don't do this because they want to be A* parents, they do this because an overtired child is an absolute nightmare to look after! Tired children just do not cope. And we, as adults, share a child's sensitivity to a shortfall of sleep.

So, start by approaching your sleep like a responsible parent and take from the wisdom of your younger self. Know that you need sleep. Know that nothing good comes from depriving yourself of it.

BED IS FOR SLEEP AND SEX ONLY

Like the good parent, you can set up your own good sleep routine. Sleep 'hygiene' consists of a set of things we can do, that lay a clear pathway for you to reach the Land of Nod. Know the following (and return to them anytime you need to):

» Good sleep loves a routine, so start getting up at the same time every day, resisting the temptation to 'catch up' on sleep on your days off.

» Avoid the daytime nap. Napping in the day is often at the expense of a proper full night's sleep.

» If you wake in the night, don't look at the time. Waking once or twice in the night is perfectly normal, but concrete knowledge of the exact time will often cause anxiety, making it harder to get back to sleep.

» If you're wide awake and sleep seems miles away, it is usually better to get up rather than stay in bed.

» Bed should be for sleep and for sex. That is it. This means no doom-scrolling and no Netflix; the blue light from screens is the enemy of our circadian rhythms.

» Cutting back on caffeine, nicotine and alcohol help with good sleep patterns.

» Take a hot bath or shower before bed and make sure your room is dark and cool (in temperature). A comfy mattress and lovely bed linen are gifts to your sleeping self.

Nourish Yourself

The relationship between our diet and our mental health is complex. We all know there is a significant link between what we put in our bodies and how we feel. Some foods can have a positive impact on mood: vegetables, pulses, grains and good-quality protein all impact on how we feel (we can't expect just to eat a nutritious diet and feel great, but as part of your maintenance it's supportive). Actively participating with the story that you are valuable, and treating your body with this sentiment, can be helpful when we think about what we put into our systems.

Foods that trick the brain into releasing chemicals into our system that we might need for a temporary kick or mood lift include things like caffeine, chocolate, sugary or salty things. These actually make it harder for us to understand and moderate our moods. They alter our state by giving us a temporary high, so it can be more difficult to notice what we are really feeling.

SIDE NOTE

It feels important to say here that we are not unpacking the very sensitive and complicated relationship some of us have with eating patterns and are not including eating disorders here which are psychoanalytically too layered to include in a top tip. We are also not discrediting the monumental struggle some of us have to maintain a positive relationship with food and alcohol. So when we apparently flippantly talk in this section about a moderate approach to intaking nutritious things, we are not without understanding and empathy for the very real struggle this is for many of us. We are also not nutritionists or dieticians. These are just some things we understand about the connection between nutrients and how we feel.

TIME FOR REFLECTION

» Do you notice when you want to reach for foods you know aren't actually great for you?

>   » Is it when you are feeling stressed, overwhelmed, upset, confused or vulnerable?
>   » Does it make any significant impact or do you just feel the benefits momentarily?

Think about those immediate distractions we might use – Netflix, wine, WhatsApp – and think about some foods doing the same for our internal systems. Saturated fats, for example, can be difficult for our systems to cope with, as they act as a block for other foods to convert into nutrients. In the same way, they act as a block to our natural emotional flow. They derail and distract the neural pathways in our brain that process emotion, so that we have momentary relief from whatever is causing us discomfort. However, our feelings don't just vanish with no attention; they lay dormant until they re-emerge, so the food hit acts as a distraction, not a solution.

We aren't suggesting totally vetoing anything that gives you a bit of comfort. Abstinence from the food and drinks we enjoy isn't always a sustainable approach, as we can end up feeling hard done by. However, think about moderation and not using these things as the sole crutch to change your mood or to block out feelings. Many clients notice changes in their eating habits at times of emotional distress; often we'll notice clients talking more about food or comfort foods when they are finding life harder, lonelier and looking for an escape.

SOME RESEARCH ABOUT FOOD AND FEELINGS

The research into how diet can help treat mental health problems is relatively new and still quite limited, but one randomised controlled trial examined the role of diet in the treatment of depression. Over 12 weeks, 67 individuals with moderate or severe depression received either dietary counselling or social support in addition to their current treatment. The dietary intervention was similar to a Mediterranean diet – lots of vegetables, fruits, whole grains, oily fish, extra virgin olive oil, legumes and raw nuts. It also allowed for some red meat and dairy. At the end of the study, those on this diet had significantly greater improvements in depression symptoms.

According to the SMILES trial (conducted with 891 women, between the ages of 45 and 65), there is an inverse relationship between fruit and vegetable consumption and recurring depressive symptoms: low fruit and veg = more depressive symptoms. The research examined the association between fruit and veg consumption and the risk of having recurring depressive symptoms over a two-year period.

The reasons behind why this is the case are unconfirmed, but several factors have been suggested. The first is that antioxidant properties within fruit and veg prevent oxidative stress on the brain, potentially reducing the incidence of depression. Another proposition is that a deficiency in the nutrients that play a significant role in neurotransmitter synthesis, such as folate, B12 and B6, could be a cause of increased depressive symptoms. In addition, stress-related disorders such as depression and anxiety have shown strong associations with dysfunction of the microbiome-gut-brain axis.

STAY HYDRATED

Take time to drink water. It's a simple and essential act of self-care. Water connects us to our primary needs: 'What do I need to keep myself alive?' It encourages flow: flow of things within the body, and connects us unconsciously to the wider flow of water in the world. The flow of water is the very antithesis to stuckness. Water can also take us out of flight, fight or freeze mode, reminding us of our ability to salivate, and provides the antidote to the dry mouth which can be a symptom of stress and anxiety.

We experience fight, flight or freeze responses involuntarily and physiologically. Changes happen in the body and mind when we feel threatened. These are ancestral responses we've inherited that were designed to keep us safe from threats, either preparing us to face them, escape or hide from danger. In today's world, these responses can be limiting. Reaching to drink some water is a reminder that we have other choices in how we respond (reaching to drink water in years gone by would not have been an option).

AIM FOR BALANCE AND MODERATION

Develop a moderate approach to the way you eat and drink. Don't go for an all-or-nothing approach or totally deny yourself things you like and that bring you joy. That's a miserable way to live and can lead to controlling behaviours. Perhaps aim for one nice coffee a day, drinking it in a more ritualistic way, where you enjoy the process and are more conscious about it. Or a couple of squares of chocolate every day to look forward to. Keeping flexible, sustainable routines around foods is useful (for example, 'every time I order a coffee or a glass of wine I'll also drink water') so that we avoid the often addictive diet cultures.

Labelling, calling or referring to foods as 'good' or 'bad' can trigger regressive feelings (back when you were not allowed sweets as a kid, or made to go to bed with no dinner if you did something wrong), which can put us into defensive, self-protection, shut down mode. This can lead to punitive thoughts and behaviours around being good or bad if we consume those certain foods. For example, 'I'm a bad person because I ate that', rather than a more compassionate, enquiring approach which might sound like, 'What were you feeling and what did you need? Gosh you poor thing, that sounds rubbish.'

It can be useful to think about what we put in our bodies as things we *need* (fresh stuff, fruit, veg, fibre, protein) and things we *want* (Haribo, salty chips), with an aim to striking a balance between the two. Be conscious whether a food choice is something you really feel you need, and/or it is something you want. Both serve a purpose, but knowing the difference can help.

Avoid binge or reward culture where you can. For example, 'I'll go full force all weekend with everything I want and then deprive myself all week to cancel it out.' When we overfill and then restrict ourselves, we are not providing a stable base for our feelings; we become preoccupied with what we are, or aren't, consuming, which can act as a defence against feeling.

TRY CONSCIOUS EATING

Notice the impact certain foods have on you. Keep a diary of what's happened in your life when you want to eat loads of things you know don't make you feel great, and also what you eat that contributes to helping you feel better. Observe your emotional patterns around food – when you crave certain things or when you lean on food and what the triggers are, so that you have a more conscious approach to what is going into your body and why.

Movement and Exercise

When we are struggling with our mental health we often feel stuck. Nothing reinforces this feeling more than staying static. When we stretch, move or change our physical position we remind ourselves subconsciously of what we are capable of. We remind our bodies that moving from one place to the next is possible. This strengthens our sense of hope and can contribute to us feeling differently. We don't all need to be athletes and we aren't suggesting that you need to try to be, but moving in a way that feels possible for you is a great activator for shifting you from one mental space into another. Doing something physical releases cortisol which helps us manage stress. Being physically active also gives your brain something to focus on, which can be a positive coping strategy for difficult times.

We spend a lot of our lives sitting at desks these days, where most things are so easily accessible with little physical effort, not experiencing the power of our bodies, and we need to counter this proactively. People often say they're too busy to exercise, that they don't have enough time, when in fact it's because they aren't prioritising themselves over other things. Start to think of exercise (in whichever form you like) as essential as opposed to desirable.

Even when it feels like the last thing you want to do, encourage yourself to do something physical in the knowledge that it will create a positive impact. Take some time out to walk in nature, to do a gentle ten-minute stretch or, if you feel you can, engage with the gym, exercise classes, online sessions, walking or running with a friend, dancing at home . . . Whatever it is – move!

We often jump to the conclusion that we don't like exercise because we've had a bad experience, perhaps felt intimidated in the gym, or feel afraid to try new things. These are valid and worth exploring, but are not actually related to the positive impact movement can and does have on your body.

No one really goes into exercise feeling like it is exactly what they want to be doing, but no one ever really regrets it afterwards. It's unlikely you'll hear someone say, 'I wish I had not exercised'. Know that the labour involved in working on your mental health isn't instantly gratifying, but all of it contributes to your resilience pot; all of the small steps add up.

Things that might help build exercise into your life in a more sustainable way include:

1. **Diarise it:** Build spaces in your day to move, and stick with those. You can block times in your diary as recurring events so that this is allocated and reserved, highlighting the importance that your body matters and, in turn, reminding you that you matter.

2. **Mix it up:** There are so many different ways to move your body, so why not try something new? Make sure you notice when exercise becomes an extension of ways you might chastise yourself or beat yourself up. Do you use your exercise routine as something rigid to measure yourself against? Chasing race times, distances run, number of burpees? Notice when exercise is not supporting self-care, but hindering it. Doing a variety of movement is good for your body and reinforces your ability to seek out and make change.

3. **Be realistic:** Avoid chastising yourself or punishing yourself for missing a workout. Set realistic targets for how often you exercise, be gentle with yourself, and re-evaluate if you don't reach them.

Harry (27) came to see us over a 16-week period. He was finding it difficult to make decisions and changes in his life. He had a fairly good self-care routine, but after several sessions, he disclosed that he ran ten miles every day, the same route at the same time. He said he hated it and he had shin splints, but he didn't feel he was able to make a change to his exercise routine. He knew the movement helped him but it had become unhelpful to his life in the way he was approaching it. This became our objective within the initial session – to make a change to his exercise routine, our belief being that if he was able to make changes in this area of his life it would potentially empower him to let go of rigidity in other areas. He started first with changing the run time, distance and then the route. We then introduced alternate days of running and yoga, which he was terrified of at first. We then reduced running to once a week, and then not at all, and he replaced it with different things (the exercise itself was helpful to his body so removing his desire to be physically active would not have been helpful). He suggested a 'bingo' day which is where he chose a random exercise every month and tried that.

It was really hard initially for him to make the changes, with feelings of grief, fear, distress and anxiety to the loss of his schedule. He was able to share his nervousness and, with support, was able to make the incremental changes. He was also able to make clear parallels to other areas of his life, expressed through the way he approached exercise. As the changes started to evolve, he became energised, excited and more relaxed in general and felt more equipped to make more significant changes in his life.

> Small changes build the blocks
> for us to make bigger ones.

Breathe

Our breath connects us to living and our ability to survive. Even at the shittiest times in your life, you are still breathing. It is the reliable, reassuring consistent thing we have to anchor to, in times of distress and overwhelm.

Your breath also give you signs about what's going on for you: is your breath fast, struggling, hyper or erratic? These all show you something about what's happening in your feeling self. When you feel at your worst, taking a moment to connect to your breath can bring you back to the reassuring, consistent and automatic nature of your body's will and ability to stay alive. You can also control your breath, which gives you a sense of mastery when you might otherwise feel without control of your feelings or life events.

A CALMING BREATH

Here is a simple breathing exercise to try when you feel a need to calm your thoughts. Why not try it now so it will become more automatic when you need it the most?

1. Lie on your back and bend your knees over a pillow, or stand still against a wall.
2. Place one hand flat against your chest and the other on your stomach.
3. Take slow, deep breaths through your nose. Keep the hand on your chest still as your stomach rises and falls with your breathing.
4. Next, exhale slowly through pursed lips. As you breathe out, feel the weight of your muscles and your bones. Visualise sinking into a giant marshmallow.
5. Repeat for as long as you wish.

Rest

Hygge, the Danish concept of valuing cosy, simple things, is great. But have you heard of the Dutch concept of Niksen – aka doing absolutely nothing? Niksen is about being idle as a form of stress relief. Appropriate activities are purposeless ones, like staring out of a window, hanging out or listening to music.

There is so much pressure culturally for us to be productive. We have become so used to filling in every minute of the day with something to do, endlessly scrolling through apps. Productivity in itself isn't bad; it's the pressure to be productive or seem busy all the time that's taking a toll on our mental health. We must begin to combat it by lessening the things we do, by embracing times in the day devoid of any activity, and letting our minds rest for a change.

I (Jodie) worked with Dola (31) for three years. Dola came to see me because she was unable to decide if she wanted to marry her partner and it was causing her to feel really distressed at her inability to find a view for the future. I noticed that she would be on her phone up until the moment she came through the doorway to the session. She appeared hyper-vigilant, quick to speak and respond, and she said she embraced the always-on culture she had at work and felt she thrived on it (I was not so sure).

After several weeks of working together, I told her that I was curious about why she was wearing flip-flops in November. She said she hadn't been able to decide what boots to buy so hadn't bought any. I asked her if her feet were cold and she took a moment to say, yes, they were actually. I suggested that most likely wasn't very nice for her and could I help her think about an alternative. This led her into saying, 'I just feel so tired all the time. I'm not sure what I want or need anymore. I can't even decide what to have for lunch.' We were then able to identify that she never took breaks in the day, she had less than six hours' sleep each night and she worked on weekends. When she did socialise, she did so with people from work.

I said that perhaps she was burnt out, which was causing her to be disconnected from her body, her self and her prevailing needs. Making choices that felt intrinsic to her wellness would, therefore, be near-on impossible. She couldn't remember the last time she did nothing, had no plans, could just be with herself and maybe her partner. Our work became focused on building in rest every day, building up to proper holiday times and embracing the fear and grief she felt about switching off. Dola had core beliefs (see page 82) around her worth being connected to her output – her father had been an academic who appeared to value her mostly when she did well. Over time she learnt to notice when she began to feel a rest was due and we built this in, enforced it, in fact. Time to do nothing. She found it challenging at first but soon looked forward to it. She got married and had two children in the time I worked with her and her indecision never presented itself in the room again. I also didn't see her in flip-flops in winter with cold feet again!

Give yourself permission to do nothing for moments in the day. Give your mind a chance to recharge and reset. Take a big breath and pause. It's like mindfulness, but instead of zoning in, you're zoning out.

Find a space in your house for Niksen, preferably with a window, or somewhere relaxing and quiet, so you can centre in, let go of all distractions and just be. Start with five minutes, then ten minutes, and work your way up to however long you want it to be, so you get back to your day refreshed and ready to go.

SIGNS THAT YOU'RE LONG OVERDUE A BREAK FROM WORK

Do you recognise any of these? Do you:

» feel exhausted, even after a good night's sleep?
» find it hard to concentrate?
» feel irritable and overly critical at work?
» lack satisfaction from your achievements?
» feel impatient with colleagues or clients?
» have unexplained headaches and stomach problems?
» find it hard to feel motivated?
» use food, drugs or alcohol to cope or numb?

Rest should not be treated as something only to be earned through overworking, overachieving and exhaustion. Rest from work says: 'I value my work and I want to offer the best I can to it.'

Know that most of our processing, repair and internal sorting out is done in the moments where we do little, where we have a chance to settle down and not think productively, or be outcome-driven. These moments of meandering are where some of our most significant growth happens.

These basics are the foundations for keeping you well enough and in good enough shape to have the capacity to process internal matter. When we are not preoccupied with needing food, sleep and movement, we have the option to do more of something else and build up proper self-care. This is a wonderful state for internal balance – when there is nothing to be done, much can happen!

Chapter 6

Proper Self-Care

We are all familiar with the idea of a face mask or a day at the spa, a cheat day or a walk in the country as components for 'self-care'. These are things we can all most likely do, without much challenge and work. We understand them as a form of self-affection or a way of telling ourselves that we matter. The real self-care, though, is much less easy, much less luxurious and much harder work, but the rewards will be longer-lasting and the impact felt much more broadly. Proper self-care is not just saying *yes* to the things that are good for us, but also saying *no* to the things that cause us harm and stunt our growth.

We know that the most effective way we can love children is by giving them boundaries within which they feel safe, giving them a mixture of encouragement and strong guidance that doesn't always feel easy on them. Think of your own self-care in the same way – proper self-care may feel tough, but once you begin you'll understand the benefits and feel them across your life.

Once we are able to embed some of the basic foundations outlined in the previous chapter into our daily lives we have the opportunity to begin building up – encouraging ourselves to think a little differently, a little deeper and more philosophically about how we are in the world, in relation to our feelings. We can begin to challenge ourselves more, look more closely at the tactics we have adopted to avoid feeling. We are going to look at the negative patterns of behaviour we can fall into, with a view to some shift and change. Below are some of the themes we hear often in the therapy room:

Remove the Mask

It has become normal to live a filtered life, to show up wearing a 'mask'. We were never with more power to filter, but with less truth and authenticity. We have so much technology and there are so many ways for us to hide – whether it's through apps, fake email addresses or permanent make-up. Couple this with living in a society that appears to value toughness, stoicism and fierce independence, which cements the idea that more vulnerable feelings are dangerous and are shameful parts of ourselves that can't be shared. We make connections on social media, we have thousands of followers, yet everyone is wearing masks of superficiality.

We can become fixated on how we present ourselves, what we say, the right camera angle, the filters and light, becoming more dependent on how this version of ourselves is received and validated, which often has no resemblance to how we actually feel. Because we meet such filtered versions of each other, we think we are the only ones who are struggling. We can feel alone in our imperfections, different, isolated in our struggles.

Over time, the filtered version of ourself grows bigger and our real self shrivels. It's addictive though, isn't it? The dopamine hits of our social media likes, tap tap tap . . . the comments about how we look, what we are wearing, how well we are seemingly doing. We flex our feelings of success or failure depending on the way others receive the filtered version we show them.

What we need for our sense of well-being is to be united in our human suffering, to hear ourselves in others' truthful stories. We need to share in how we are really feeling. To then see that also in others' sad, overwhelmed eyes, how they are or aren't coping with the crap life throws at us all. This is how we feel less alone, how we feel validated, seen, heard and connected for being who we are and feeling how we feel. This is a key ingredient for how we grow, how we relate and how we become more ourselves. Being able to recognise and share our own, and be with others' humanness, is a powerful, reparative and connecting experience.

Donald Winnicott, the renowned child psychotherapist, famously said, 'it's a joy to be hidden and disaster not to be found'. He's talking about the emotional crisis we will face if we keep ourselves hidden at all costs. If we think about the game of hide-and-seek on page 79, without that often joyous, trepid moment when we are actually found, the game would be joyless, meaningless. We would remain alone, unconnected, hidden. If we've been hidden too long, we might squeak or rustle in the hope of being found. For our better mental health we need to squeak more!

I (Jodie) went to watch a brilliant strategist speak about her craft. There were hundreds of people in the audience, expectantly waiting to learn something. When she began I was fidgeting and not really listening – I felt disengaged and unimpressed – and then she stopped fairly suddenly, paused and said quietly, humbly: 'I feel so anxious and overwhelmed right now. I'm worried I'm going to mess this up and disappoint you all and I really don't want that to happen.' At that moment I could totally relate, engage and feel connected to her. She went on to deliver something brilliant. I felt completely at ease in seeing her for herself and reassured that it mattered to her so much. It meant something to us both. I found meaning in her truth and she was able to connect with us, giving her the confidence to continue. She allowed us to see under her mask.

TIME FOR REFLECTION

Encourage yourself to share where you are at and what's happening for you, unfiltered. Try small steps at first, in safe relationships and environments. Share what you are really feeling, even if it isn't concise and neat like an Insta catchphrase. Authentically and truthfully share your reality and see how that feels:

» 'I am really struggling with the kids at the moment; I just can't seem to connect with them.'

» 'I was really nervous about seeing you today because ...'

>   » 'It felt really hard for me to commit to this plan . . .'
>   » 'I don't think I've been looking after myself very well.'
>   » 'I haven't really wanted to see anyone or do anything.'
>   » 'I feel a bit out of control with my spending/drinking/ sex life.'
>   » 'I am not feeling good about my body and it's making me feel . . .'
>   » 'Can I ask for your advice about something that's upsetting me?'

Of course, this can feel risky. There is a risk of being judged, of being invalidated, of not being heard, but the risk far outweighs the alternative, which is to stay alone and hidden. To feel safe, secure and deeply connected to others is an essential part of the human experience.

BE MORE BEEGU . . .

Beegu is a beautiful book by Alexis Deacon. It tells the story of a rabbit-like alien who's stranded on Earth. She is lost and wandering. She fails to make contact with the strange creatures she encounters: animals don't seem to understand her, windblown leaves won't stay still to listen, and adults can't hear her. Lost and alone, she wants to give up. But at last, on a school playground when she is feeling at her most vulnerable and alone, she is able to shine her light and connect with a group of children. Her spirits are lifted, she radiates and her mother ship is able to find her light. She is heard and found.

There is something really resonating in the story of Beegu and it describes an important metaphor, which is that sometimes, when you feel at your most hopeless, when all your defences are down, you are able to reach out with real meaning to others. When you stop pretending and show your true self, you are able to feel less alone.

TIME FOR REFLECTION

Have you ever had an experience when you've felt at your most wretched, most lost and without the energy to hold on to the mask? What does it feel like when you do drop the mask of having it all together? When you ask a friend to lend you money because you're struggling, when you ask someone to hold your hand when you go to the hospital or pick you up after an awful day at work? What is it like when you tell someone you aren't eating properly, or are drinking too much, or feel like a bad parent? What does it feel like for you when you show people what's really going on for you?

We often wait until we are at rock bottom to let people in. Try to consciously invite people into your life, in a way that feels more authentic, sooner, rather than waiting until you need help desperately. Proactively invite more Beegu-style connections, more often. This can look like and sound like:

» WhatsApping a friend or sending them a voice note to let them know how your day really is.

» Setting up informal check-ins with your line manager.

» Asking to take a walk with someone.

» Sharing with someone what's making you angry, happy, sad . . .

» Asking for help with more everyday things.

» Sharing school drop-off/pick-ups with another parent.

» Being more honest about what is imperfect about your life.

Say No to Busy

Busyness can be addictive and/or habitual. It can be a fear-based response to trauma that keeps us apart from the feelings we'd be forced to acknowledge if we slowed down. Trauma can be related to anything we find difficult to process, integrate or internalise, or when an event, or series of events, causes us a lot of stress. This could be parental separation, being fired from your job or struggling through an acrimonious divorce. Perhaps you feel constantly misunderstood or minimised. Maybe you have experienced your fair share of let-downs. Trauma can be subtle; it's not always a huge event, but it will be something we are unconsciously trying to avoid.

THINGS THAT MIGHT KEEP YOU BUSY

» overcommitting

» fear of letting people down

» being seen as boring

» fear of what people will say if you say no

» feeling obligated, in rescuer mode

> » your parents/caregivers were always busy (learnt behaviour)
> » avoidance of feelings (such as grief, anger, distress)
> » feeling disconnected to ourselves
> » unhappiness
> » fear of being alone
> » avoiding difficult conversations
> » challenging relationships (for example, with kids, family, partners)
> » avoidance of things that might help us stay well (such as exercise, rest, eating well)

Busyness has become a culturally acceptable avoidance strategy. Our default response to difficult things is to look for something to distract us. We unconsciously do anything we can to keep busy and away from what we can't face. When we stop and slow down, it can get very uncomfortable. How often do you get poorly when you go on holiday? Or feel worse at the weekend when you aren't working? Or afraid if you have a weekend without plans?

Unpopular opinion: hustle culture is fucking us up.

Allowing times of nothingness is precious because it's how we stay connected. It stops us from burying old emotions which actually need to be acknowledged and nurtured.

The tendency to move, speak and think fast, to be occupied with multiple tasks, to have a never-ending to-do list, to be always on the go, and to be relentlessly busy as a way of life, serves a purpose that doesn't speak to our well-being. Things busyness does:

» **It acts as a defence against feeling.** All the while we are doing, doing, doing, we don't feel so much. We do not give ourselves a chance to notice how we might be feeling. Therefore we defend against what might be difficult or painful. We hide and can sometimes be lost behind our busyness. Busyness can be a strategy for getting through the day without having to feel the unresolved trauma that lives in our bodies as pain, grief, anxiety, fear and anger. But equally, it keeps us apart from feelings of joy.

» **It helps us feel a false sense of purpose.** All the while we are doing tasks, moving from one thing to the next, we are attached to, and identified with, our *doing* and not our *being*. Being busy can be mistaken and internalised as fulfilling a purpose.

» **It hides our loneliness.** If we are busy being popular or needed, we are serving others or tasks. We make ourselves indispensable and this can feel like not being alone. If we remove our 'doing' we can feel very vulnerable. Busyness and being over-attached to the service of others is a mechanism for control against loss: 'All the while I serve this purpose and do this for them they can't leave me.'

» **It makes us feel glamorous.** We celebrate busyness as a culture. We can wrongly believe that those who are busy are somehow more in demand, more useful, more popular than us, and it can make us crave that. This can validate our busyness and lead us away from a more restful space, which could be much more nourishing and useful for our well-being.

» **It adds to our stress levels.** There is no dancing around this: being busy is stressful. It might feel energising at the time, and we can feel motivated by a bit of stress, but over long periods and without consciousness to it, it really adds to our feelings of being overwhelmed and contributes to a deep sense of fatigue. It also means that we often do things half-heartedly. We aren't actually able to arrive at one thing before we are leaving for the next. So it gives us a chance to do nothing very well. We might have a constant sense of not doing things well enough, or doing lots but finding little meaning, going through the motions. We then feel less energised and more depleted by things.

Moving fast and doing multiple tasks keeps the trauma pattern in place. In order to shift the pattern, we have to do something different. We have to be willing to build our capacity to slow down, to come back into a relationship with being and feeling, rather than doing, doing, doing.

TIME FOR REFLECTION

Practise slowing down by allocating windows to stop and just be. This might be for five or ten minutes at first, and then you can build this up slowly.

» Encourage yourself to have fewer or no plans at certain times, even if this feels really frightening and uncomfortable.

» Practise things which bring you to yourself, for example, reading (although be careful that reading isn't a way to distract yourself through learning or doing) or drawing.

» Allow yourself to just rest. Resting is for just that – resetting and connecting to yourself. Don't use this time to add more bullet points to your to-do list.

» Notice any fear feelings that creep in at times that feel slow; notice their discomfort and feel them anyway. When we have become used to 'busy', anything else can feel fear-inducing, unknown, uncertain and different. Allow your vulnerabilities a space to be felt and lean into a different pace and space.

When we allow ourselves to slow down and fully feel whatever's there, we work to process and dissolve old emotions. We don't allow them to scare us away from ourselves anymore.

SIGNS YOUR BODY IS TELLING YOU TO REST

» You have jaw, neck and/or shoulder tension.

» You're tired, even after a good sleep.

» It's hard to focus.

» You've been losing hair.

» Your eating patterns have changed.

» You've got an upset stomach for no reason.

- » You find it hard to fall or stay asleep.
- » You're getting colds/your immune system is run down.
- » Your chest is tight and you have headaches.
- » Making decisions, big or small, is a challenge.

BFF Your Inner Child

This idea of 'best friending' the you from your childhood has become a kind of therapy cliché, a bit like wearing socks and sandals and burning sage at yoga (both excellent as it turns out). Many of us find the idea a bit cheesy. Most likely this is born from people's fear of what it might mean to spend some time on the younger version of themselves and what this might bring up. It can feel scary, intimidating and upsetting. It might risk destabilising your view of your family or your past, which in itself can feel like something to be avoided. Most things that get mocked are because they pose a threat to some aspect of our safety, but safe doesn't always encourage growth. 'Inner child' work brings us in to contact with aspects that might challenge our perception of things and rock the boat a little.

We are always careful of how we introduce inner child work in the therapy room, not wanting it to make people run a mile. So we'll do the same here and urge you to keep an open mind and quieten down your possible resistance, where you can. Inner child work can be pure magic for your growth and change; it can be hard and uncomfortable, but growing often is.

Your inner child is your original or true self before systemic and environmental experiences impacted you. It is the original core of who you are. You might find it's a more carefree, playful, creative, silly, cheeky, inquisitive, quiet version of yourself. It's possible that a younger version of you was more connected to your truth in an uninhibited way. Finding ways to reconnect to that version of yourself can be revitalising, energising and liberating. It can help us be less judgemental of ourselves and more accepting. Finding ways to reconnect with your inner child is an important part of making contact with what's really happening for you.

Your inner child doesn't refer to that part of your brain dedicated solely to childish thoughts. Nor does it mean the more childish behaviours you might inhabit sometimes. The inner child often speaks loudest when you are faced with challenges or emotional disturbance in your life. The inner child reflects the child you once were, both the good and the less good bits.

Learning to take your inner child seriously, and to consciously communicate with that little being within you – to listen to how they feel and what they need now – is a powerful tool in growing through what you've been through. We can't expect our adult selves to be healed if we don't go back and visit our inner child. We might be able to patch things up, but we can't fully repair them if we aren't able to connect with our younger selves.

The needs of your inner child might be much the same as your adult self: love, acceptance, protection, nurture and understanding. If you didn't sufficiently receive these in the past from your parents or caregivers, you need to go back and provide a little of what was needed then. What was done cannot be undone, but you can go back and try to look it in the face. Accept the painful bits and celebrate the joyous ones.

You can take care of and celebrate your inner child's needs *now* to support how you feel.

WAYS TO BEFRIEND YOUR INNER CHILD

1. **Remind yourself.** Look through old pictures of yourself and see what it feels like: what do you think or feel about what you see? What do you remember about when the picture was taken? What was happening in your life, what was or wasn't working, and how does that make you feel? Were your needs being met at that time or not? How does thinking about it make you feel?

2. **Write yourself a letter.** Write your younger self a letter. Give yourself some advice that your adult self knows. Extend, in your letter, love, care and attention to your younger self, offering them the things they might have needed back then. Allow yourself the luxury of giving yourself what you need most.

3. **Play.** What things did you enjoy as a child? Think about the activities, games and creative things you used to do. Find ways to do them again. For example, painting, craft, dancing or Lego. Which places did you enjoy going to – playgrounds or places you walked in or holidays you had? Can you revisit any of them? Did you have hobbies or collect things and can you find ways of recapturing that?

4. **Close your eyes and visualise the 'little you'.** Form a dialogue. Ask questions like 'What are you feeling, what do you need right now?' and 'How can I support you?'

5. **Notice what feelings you are connected to.** Are you able to find a more unfiltered, more authentic version of yourself back there? Maybe you have uncovered some wounds you had ignored and some glorious things you had forgotten about yourself.

Say No to Too Many Experts and Self-Help Shit

As we write this we are aware of the irony of what we are saying! There is a huge amount of content available in the self-help space. Other people's opinions, views and ideas around *your* mental health are readily available. Suggestions about what you should and should not be doing can be found almost everywhere you look. Friends telling you what they feel you should do, others sharing what they've been doing and what works for them, the shoulds and should nots . . . These can feel endless and, when you are looking for answers, you will find them almost anywhere you look.

Flooding yourself with too much theory, too many tasks, too many ideas around your own mental health can actually make you feel *more* disconnected from what is actually happening for you, and what you need. You can become so focused on what you should/could/must be doing/thinking/feeling, that you are not truly able to listen to yourself. It can act as a defence against your own feelings. If you are feeling overloaded with other people's ideas and opinions, it might stop you from connecting to yourself and what you really need.

TIME FOR REFLECTION

» Do you think you might be overwhelmed by advice, however well-intentioned? How can you cut through all the noise and find meaning that's helpful to you?

» Keep a notebook or scrapbook of images, quotes or references that mean something to you. Don't fixate on them, but know they are there to refer to.

» When something does speak to you, or you become very interested in a view or opinion around self-help, try to dig a bit deeper about *why* it speaks to you. Reflect on what it can reveal about where you are at and what you are going through. Don't keep it at a distance – bring it closer towards you and your reality.

» Notice when you are hiding in other people's views and try to find your own voice about how you are feeling. Ask 'Am I learning or hiding here?'

The ideas in this chapter are an invitation for you to challenge your beliefs around what self-care really means to you. To reframe self-care in a way that opens up the opportunity for challenge, care and ideas for when you find that yet another face mask really isn't making you feel any better. We hope you can start to consider self-care as preventative and action-based, as opposed to reactive. Bath bombs, massages, that pint of beer or glass of fizz don't really help you to resolve anything; they might act as a balm for when you are working on yourself, but they do not have any lasting effecting on your mental health. Proper self-care is much less Instagrammable.

Chapter 7

Routines and Rituals

Rituals provide us with a daily opportunity to structure our lives, to give us containment when we need it. They enable us to practise proper self-care. They are not to be confused with extra jobs to do or things to busy you with, but as soothing, useful acts that can support your well-being. No one needs more shit to do that feels like a task, but we feel these mental maintenance routines and rituals are worth it. More energy is used up when you avoid or ignore yourself and your feelings – it is much more productive to be proactive.

You might notice that when life feels challenging, holding on to routines and rituals that support you can feel difficult. This is the time when we need them most; routines and rituals can anchor us to ourselves and help us when we feel adrift in life. We often ask our clients what they did today, this week, to take care of themselves, and most will look back at us sheepishly or worried and say 'nothing'.

So what do we class as a ritual within the mental mainte-nance framework? We consider rituals as things that you do often and regularly as part of the work you do on your mental health. The process of conducting and completing rituals can provide us with a sense of continuity, stability and comfort amidst the constantly changing and sometimes chaotic world we live in.

Rituals provide an anchor in rough seas. We each have the resources already within us based upon our lived routines to create our own rituals to bring comfort, order and even harmony to our existence. We might find keeping rituals and routines particularly hard when we are struggling, but reaching out for them and trying to return to them can bring us hope and a sense of reassurance.

TIME FOR REFLECTION

» What was your experience of routines and rituals from childhood? Did you have a mealtime, holiday or a homework routine?

» What could you rely on as always happening?

» Are there any routines/rituals you wish you'd had?

» Have you carried any over into your adult life?

» Which routines do you like and which ones do you dread?

» Have you created any new ones that feel supportive?

» Think about your current routines and rituals. What changes could you make to them to better support yourself?

Rituals are about assigning and setting aside quality time. They are about claiming space for something that matters, so we can create a place to meet ourselves and the world with clarity, intention and meaning, even if it is just to conduct the ritual. The stirring of a cup of tea, writing in a journal, saying a prayer, making the bed, quiet words with a loved one who has died, calling someone to keep you company while you cook, lighting a candle in remembrance, that same shower playlist, therapy, a repeated walk . . . in their dailyness, these things are drenched in ceremony.

Through the practice of each of these things, we can be more present, find more order when we are overwhelmed, practise self-compassion and find a little hope in our ability to remember the familiar.

What follows are some of our ideas around rituals and positive habit-forming that might inspire you. These are by no means exhaustive.

Journal

Keep a journal that is just for you and your thoughts. It's useful to have a place to offload some of what is coming up for you; journaling helps us to get closer to our unfiltered selves. Even if it does feel like a chore at first, stay with it. It can feel like just another something to do, but really it helps our mental mainte-nance process. Write in your journal in a way that is unfiltered, giving yourself a really solid chance of hearing yourself. When we are not under pressure to write for an audience or with the anxiety of a deadline or outcome, we can be more uncensored

and less concerned with making sense, and more connected
to telling our truth. Journaling creates a space for creativity,
reflection and mindfulness, and helps us to practise 'presentee-
ism' – being with what is happening in the here and now.

There are some steps you can take to support your journaling experience, and we have included some Journal Prompts
and Time for Reflection boxes throughout the book that can
help to start you off, but really just write . . .

» You might want to write about what is happening for you
  in your life today. What does it remind you of? Does it feel
  familiar or new? Notice emerging patterns in your writing.
» It can be useful to read your writing back, to give space for
  reflection. What do you notice about what you read? How
  can you treat what you read with compassion and not judgement and see it as a way to understand yourself more?
» Honour your thoughts and feelings in your writing.
  Continuous flow is often useful, so just keep on writing
  and writing, without thinking about sentences or paragraph
  structure. Just write what comes up for you. You can use
  the technique of 'free association'; this means letting your
  mind wander and make connections with what has just been
  written or thought. Celebrate chaos, messiness and incoher-
  ence in your writing; you are not looking for a well-crafted
  essay but something that has meaning for you.
» Give yourself a set time to write if that is useful, and hold
  yourself to the routine. Remember, mental maintenance isn't
  easy – know that you may not want to do it, but go ahead
  anyway! Be realistic – five to ten minutes is a good place to
  start. You may want to set a timer.

» Use sentence props that start with 'I' when you can, such as:
   > 'I think . . .'
   > 'I feel . . .'
   > 'I am reminded of . . .'
   > 'I can/I could . . .'

You can read back what you've written at any time and, if you feel comfortable, you can also take your journal to therapy to explore with your therapist.

Listen to Your Dreams

We all know that dream interpretation can be a sketchy, fairground, mystic space, with plenty of room for disbelief and magical thinking. However, if we think about dreams personally, as being a bridge between our conscious and unconscious mind, a passage for the unspoken, unthought parts of ourselves, we can be a little more encouraging and gentle with them. Our dreams can act as a way of trying to switch on the light for us, when we might be a little in the dark. Our dreams can support us to find solutions to problems and challenges we might be facing, bringing into the light those anxieties, feelings or ideas we might have been avoiding or denying. They are little messengers, and if we tend to them they can be really quite helpful.

Dreams can leave us feeling weird, out of sorts; they might leave a resonance of deeper feelings on waking and sometimes feel a bit ominous. They might not make full sense, yet they feel somehow familiar. They might take us to darker places within ourselves, bring us into contact with people we need to speak with, or remind us of our past that can show us something. Dreams are uncensored, unlike our conscious mind, so nothing can be hidden within them. They highlight warnings and 'look outs' for us, bringing our attention to what might be needed in our conscious life.

Dreams also help us self-regulate and balance. Jung, a psychotherapist who was a massive believer in the psychological power of dreams, observed that 'dreams are driven by a natural tendency to bring resolution and closure to unfinished emotional and mental problems of the day'. Sometimes the messages are obvious or sometimes they need us to work on them; they might need to be taken to therapy, drawn or written down. They might keep repeating until we take notice.

What's useful for us is if we give our dreams a little conscious airtime and allow them to live a little in our waking lives. Make space for your dreams, invite them in, but don't try to make concrete sense of them in a linear way. Consider that there may be more than one idea or outcome for your dream, and perhaps lots of messages within it. It can be unhelpful to try to interpret your dreams too intently, but some simple steps can invite you into a bit more curiosity about what is happening for you and shed a little light on where you might need it.

When I (Jodie) started my training as a therapist some 17 years ago, I began having a repeated dream which found me in an old pub in my hometown, a grubby old man's pub with 1970s swirly carpets. It was a place that my family frequented and it was somewhere I found unstylish and a bit unpredictable and menacing. I was about 11 in the dream, running away from something up the staircase

inside the pub. At the top of the stairs I found the toilet.
I ran in, slammed the door closed and sat on the loo
to take a breath. I didn't know what I was running away
from exactly, but I knew it felt scary and at this point I
thought I'd escaped.

I sat for a moment on the loo, before I looked up
towards the old-fashioned toilet system with a pull
chain, only to be greeted by a version of my own face
hanging upside down with the chain around my neck.
I had a green suffocated face and I couldn't speak;
I was kind of gasping, trying to say something. It was
a horrid dream and it kept repeating. On waking I
wanted to leave those thoughts in my sleep, but the
recurring nature of the dream drew me back to take
notice of it, which I feel I did in some way over the
following weeks.

It felt to me that I was running away from a version
of myself that was afraid to speak, that was silenced,
and running from adult complexities I didn't understand.
I felt my dream was telling me that I couldn't escape
myself or my past, but that I could make contact with the
silenced parts of myself and listen to the more frightened,
vulnerable, less sure parts or myself, before I pushed them
down the toilet.

Once I made a little space to connect with those
ideas and feelings, which felt pretty horrid at the time, I
was able to meet my younger self with a little compassion
and allowed in some new thoughts and ideas about my
own past rather than strangling them away. That dream
eventually stopped. I did see the green version of me

again, but she was less green and less hanging and she could speak! In fact, she often appears in my dreams when it would serve me to go back and reflect on something from my past. She draws me in.

TIME FOR REFLECTION

A useful way of connecting to your dreams is to keep a notebook by your bed; use it only for dreams. Call it your dream book. Being so purposeful in the intent of listening to your dreams gives you a clear signal to yourself that you are ready and open to listening. Here are some tips to help you:

» When you wake up, write your dreams down as you remember them. Write down the key moments that stood out to you. Think about any symbols that were clear, such as water, a road, a car, old house, mum/ dad/boss, and make a list of them.

» Write down what feelings you had, for example, fear, joy or confusion.

» Before you start to interpret, free-associate with what you remember and have a play around with what your dream might be showing you. Notice what makes most sense to you. Make a list of what you associate with the key symbols you picked out - for example, water could be holiday or a fear of swimming. What sense can you make of them with regard to what's happening in your life?

» Challenge yourself to be a bit uncomfortable. Try to reveal to yourself what you would rather not, for example, 'I probably am avoiding speaking to my dad and really need to.'

» Don't be too fixated on the ideas you come up with. Let them go if they don't fit, but notice how the thought of an interpretation makes you feel: does it help you feel calmer, throw you into action, make you go: 'Ah, that makes sense?'

» Try not to use your dreams to fit your own narrative about yourself, for example, 'It's showing me I'm useless or never going to meet anyone.' Try to have a more 'zoomed out' approach to your dreams.

Being open to your dreams is a really powerful routine to include in your everyday mental maintenance. It might feel very abstract at first, but anything that challenges you into more self-awareness, more consciousness, and different ways of listening to yourself, can only support your growth and well-being.

Set Boundaries

Setting boundaries is hard work, but they are essential to healthy relationships – this includes relationships with others, with ourselves and with work. We often don't set them because we fear what others will think of us. We fear missing opportunities, we want to be seen as 'yes' people, we fear rejection and abandonment, we fear confrontation and conflict, and we

dread feeling guilty. If we set boundaries little and often, positive habit-forming around setting them can feel much more
everyday than the mountain they can sometimes seem.

We cannot expect people to place value on us if we do not
demonstrate that we value ourselves enough to hold uncomfortable
boundaries. The way you treat yourself is a marker for how others
treat you. If you value yourself, your energy, time and love, then
others are more likely to. If others watch you placing value over
your energies and time, being considerate to yourself in how you
make your decisions, they are less likely to take advantage of you,
and more likely to respect the regard you hold for yourself.

TIME FOR REFLECTION

» Do you need to set more boundaries?

» Do you feel stuck on a treadmill of overcommitment?

» Ask yourself: 'Am I doing all of this because I want to
or need to? Or am I doing all of this out of compulsion or fear? Am I doing all of this because I want
to please others over myself?'

» What is the gain to you in *not* setting boundaries?

» Do you often say 'yes' but mean 'no' and then feel
resentful, or spend ages wondering how to cancel
or pull out (driving anxiety)?

We consider setting boundaries as a ritual. Setting boundaries
takes daily practice; being repeated often makes it more likely
this will become a positive feature in your life. If we leave setting
boundaries to only times of overwhelm or crisis, or times that

are emotionally charged, we might find we aren't as good at it or it feels too scary. You cannot beat being well versed at setting and maintaining boundaries. It will only serve you for the better.

If you feel like you often betray your own needs for others, over-listen to other people's beliefs or ideas, worry about being criticised, feel afraid of feeling guilty or falling out, feel like others are treating you disrespectfully or without compassion and not saying anything, it's probably time for you to think about your boundaries.

SEVEN SUBTLE SIGNS YOU ARE PEOPLE-PLEASING

You've heard of fight, flight or freeze, but have you heard of 'fawning'? In a nutshell, it is the use of people-pleasing to diffuse conflict, feel more secure in relationships and earn the approval of others by essentially mirroring the imagined expectations and desires of other people.

1. If you're a fawn type, you're likely very focused on showing up in a way that makes those around you feel comfortable. In more toxic relationships, you might use fawning to avoid conflict. However, if no one sees your authentic self, it can lead to feelings of being misunderstood, and even resenting the fact that no one really 'sees' you.

2. Fawn types are almost always stretched thin. Eager to please others, we quickly jump to saying 'yes!' to anything that is asked of us, even if we don't want to.

3. Wanting to make those closest to us happy, we often don't share when things are really shit for us. We might let it all build up and only speak up when we're completely overwhelmed and unable to cope.

4. You might find yourself getting angry at someone, but then very quickly quash it by justifying their behaviour and pushing down your own feelings. When we suppress our own emotions to appease another, we're fawning.

5. We're trying to anticipate someone else's happiness because, deep down, we feel responsible for it – and are trying everything in our power to ensure that the people we care about aren't disappointed.

6. You might think of yourself as being agreeable and easy to get along with, but with a closer look, you might notice you're a little too agreeable. If you find yourself sitting on the fence so as not to upset anyone, you're likely fawning to some degree. Notice if you want to continue to do so.

7. If you are trying to name how you feel, but are getting caught up in a complex tangle of guilt, anger, fear and anxiety, it's likely that you have disassociated from your primary emotional responses. The less we have distinct feelings of our own, the easier it is to adapt to and accommodate the emotions of other people.

Boundaries don't have to be barriers or brick walls. They can be pliable, meshy membranes that compassionately mark out the edges of our capacity while letting others see how we like to be treated. Don't use the idea of a boundary to reinforce your own resistances. Use them to deepen relationships, to show up more authentically, help you have control over what matters in your life, and contribute to you feeling less violated or used up.

Boundaries are complicated, particularly if we are new to them. They might sound like:

» 'I would really like to be there, but I can't this week.'
» 'I'm sorry, I don't do meetings before 8am.'
» 'I don't often WhatsApp after 9pm – the afternoon is better for me.'
» 'I am happy to speak on the phone at X o'clock.'
» 'I can feel you're struggling right now. I can help by X but I can't Y.'
» 'My energy just won't stretch to that this week.'
» 'Thank you for thinking of me, but no.'
» 'I don't often go out in the week as I really need my sleep.'
» 'That's not something I am going to be able to do; I'm aware that might feel disappointing.'
» 'That doesn't work for me, but we could X instead.'
» 'Could we book another time to talk about this that works better?'
» 'I would rather you didn't include me in that group.'

HOW TO SET YOUR OWN BOUNDARIES

Start by defining what is most important to you: time, energy, rituals, relationships (if so, which ones?).

» What are you losing to lost boundaries (that exercise class, a book that needs reading, that walk in the park)? What impact does this have on you?

» Look at the bigger picture. What do you see as common themes in your life which look like you are not holding boundaries (overspending, late nights, saying yes and meaning no, agreeing to do things you do not have the capacity for)?

» How does that make you feel?

» If you feel confused about when to introduce a boundary, buy more time ('Let me think about it and get back to you', 'I'm not sure I can let you know now, I just need to check about that and I'll get back to you').

» Practise saying no. Notice any grief, fear or anxiety that saying no brings up for you. Try to live through that experience to what's on the other side. Doing this and surviving and showing up as ourselves in relation to another, often gives a more secure sense of our worth, for example, 'I am not just loved for doing what they want/need/ask. I'm still lovable when I am not in service to another.'

» Know that holding boundaries sometimes does not immediately feel good. You might feel unsafe, anxious, confused or alone at first. This is the jumping from one lily pad to the other moment. Where are you going to land? Most often it is closer to where you want to be, so let the period of uncertainty breathe a little and sit with the discomfort.

» Know that just because a boundary is set once, it doesn't mean it's done and dusted – you might need to return to it over and over with the same person. Habits are hard to break.

» As painful as it is coming into contact with our limitations, sharing them with others only strengthens relationships.

» If your boundaries cannot be respected or regarded by others, try to understand why, and then make a decision about what that means for your relationship.

SIDE NOTE

If you have an ulterior motive other than your own self-preservation to saying no, then try to own that. For example, withdrawing your love or time as an act of punishment or for attention is not 'setting boundaries' – it's more likely avoiding conflict, triggered behaviour, or something else playing out. Don't mistake misdirecting anger, rage or meanness with boundaries.

Face Up to Money

Money is such a powerful and often emotional subject, which is why understanding our emotional relationship with it can be particularly helpful in maintaining our mental health. We project meaning on to money, effectively 'loading' it with feelings around security and control, using it as a barometer for how successful or not we are, pitting ourselves against others. We do not talk about money enough, and it is one of the biggest contributors to poor mental health and feelings of loneliness, stress and overwhelm. If we can encourage ourselves to talk about money more frequently, whether you have lots or a little, with less pressure and more honesty, it'll become more everyday, and less shame-, fear- and anxiety-causing. Worrying about talking about money for fear of what others will think of us, or how they'll view us, can enforce us to keep complicated feelings about our relationship with money inside, which can feel lonely and isolating. Establishing a ritual where you talk more often about money, and your feelings and experiences around it, and/or face up to and organise your finances, rather than not looking at them, can support your growth.

TIME FOR REFLECTION

»   What are your feelings about your own financial situation?
»   What's your relationship to money?
»   How do you feel about money and other people?
»   What was the relationship to money in your own family? What was the story that was told about money in your family? Was it one of caution? One of abundance? One of betrayal or conflict? One of scarcity? Of stability, instability?
»   How do you view work and money?

There are a few ways that we can characterise our feelings towards money. Some of us are very cautious: unwilling to spend money on anything unless we absolutely have to, and we squirrel the rest away. Some of us love to spend money and will spend every last penny – even if it would be more sensible to slow down and keep some for the end of the month or a rainy day. Most of us are somewhere in the middle, sometimes spending lots or treating ourselves, other times in a season of saving.

Generally, how our relationship with money has developed can be traced back to our upbringing. We tend to acquire our feelings, thoughts and ideas around money from the people we spend the most time with growing up – our parents or care-givers. In some cases, we might mirror our parents' or caregivers' relationship with money. If our parents were overly cautious with money, we might take this as a lesson and do the same thing. However, it can also mean we do the opposite. Sometimes, we might try to provide our own kids, partners or ourselves with what we never had, so someone who grew up with very little money or with strict parents might be lavish with gifts and see spending as a way of allowing for an experience that was never had.

In our relationships, we can also 'act out' roles, mirroring the parent–child dynamic with one as 'provider' and the other as 'provided for'. Both roles can have a deeply significant impact on our emotions, feeding into our sense of security.

A progressive and actionable step when it comes to improving our relationship to finances is simply talking honestly about it. The more our thoughts, fears, envies and stories stay locked in around money, the more toxic it becomes. Talk about money: with your partner, colleagues, family and friends. Demystify it.

Talk about how you *feel* about it, what it brings up for you, what it reminds you of, what the story of it was in your family, what it meant for you in the past, what it means for you right now and what it means for you in the future.

TIME FOR REFLECTION

» Could you talk with your friends or partner about money?

» Share when you're struggling.

» Share when you're spending too much.

» Make it one of your self-care check-ins with friends/ trusted people.

Try Therapy

Many of you might feel that therapy is for other people, for people with more troubles or a bigger trauma than you, for others who seem less 'well' than you. This is a common misconception about therapy and one that prevents loads of people from accessing it. Therapy should be a place where you can be celebrated at your best, challenged at your worst and supported at your most vulnerable. It gives you a space to share with someone else the most shameful, raw, confusing parts of who you are, without judgement. It gives you a chance to practise things in a safe place that might be helpful in your life. It gives you the opportunity to voice those conversations or ideas that feel too scary for the real world initially – here you can test them out without the risk. You can say what you feel, get cross, get upset and act as you do outside the room without the ramifications or repeated cycles you might find yourself in. In the therapy room, you can be supported to enquire deeply about why you are behaving in the way you are, in order to try to make sense of it.

Traditional reasons why you might begin therapy:

» You're stressed, and everything you feel is intense.
» You've suffered a trauma, and you can't stop thinking about it.
» You have unexplained and recurrent headaches, stomach aches or a run-down immune system.
» You're using a substance to cope.
» You're feeling rubbish.
» You feel disconnected from previously loved activities.
» Your relationships are strained (inside or outside of work).
» Your friends have told you they're concerned.

Other (equally valid) reasons you might go to therapy, from a 'wellness' perspective:

» You want to thrive in your career.
» You want to make good relationships great.
» You want to understand your purpose (inside and outside of work).
» You want to find balance.

» You want to connect with your creativity.
» You want some scaffolding to maintain high performance.
» You want a place to practise for real life.
» You want an hour each week to focus on yourself.

Therapy is also a place of affirmation and a good therapist will offer a container for your story to unfold. Here, you have the opportunity to process what happened in your life. The way you tell your story, the pace at which you tell it and the details you include can all be really meaningful when you have a chance to explore them. When stories are spoken, release happens. What is locked and stored in the body can be let out. The speaking of the previously unspeakable, in a space where we feel heard, seen and understood – this is therapy.

I can remember when I (Jodie) arrived in therapy for the first time, 18 years ago. I took a taxi and made it wait outside in case I wanted to escape quickly. I'm pretty sure I kept my sunglasses on for the entire session and I spent most of it trying to convince the therapist of all the reasons I didn't need to be there, even though I had taken myself there willingly. It was such a strange experience and I found the idea of leaving knowing nothing about my therapist really strange. I had so many questions: did she have kids, was this her house? For a while it became a really good story I told about myself at parties, joking about the experience. I returned week after week, in fact for seven years, to the same person and slowly, slowly I was able to settle down and experience the space as a place where my sunglasses were not needed.

The work of psychotherapy is to acknowledge, bear and put into perspective those feelings that have been unbearable. Despite the quick-fix, life-changing, fast-tracking solutions we are sold, this is the work. Everything else is secondary.

Within the relationship with your therapist, you can explore what might be unconsciously driving you, think about things you are doing, saying and feeling that might not be serving you, so that you can have more choices in how you live, your relationships and ultimately how you feel. A good therapist will help you see more clearly everything you are saying and also everything you aren't.

Therapy is an opportunity for you to look in a mirror and to see things that might have been unseeable to you before. It helps you shine a light on things that have been in the dark – with someone helping you to make sense of what you see. Therapy should be a place that is inviting and accepting of your mess, and a place where you can begin to sort through it in order to make sense of yourself and the world around you in a useful way. It's a place for you to be with someone else who has continued positive regard for you so that you can repair your history and prepare for your future. It's a place where you can be less alone.

A note from one of our clients on their experience of therapy: 'The profound effect of our conversations has been surprising for me. Your delicate touch has not gone unnoticed and how you managed to tease

out of me thoughts I had long banished to
the nether regions of my mind was genius.'

Think of therapy as sharing the load. We are big fans of the metaphor in the book *The Huge Bag of Worries* by Virginia Ironside,
which is a story about a little girl who carries her worries with
her in a massive bag wherever she goes. These worries include
her pet dog having fleas, that she was getting too fat and that her
best friend is moving away. We see the little girl's bag becoming
larger and heavier as it is filled with more and more worries. The
bag gets so big the girl can no longer carry it, she can't do her
normal everyday things including going to school. But she refuses
to let anyone see inside – including herself. She believes that
opening the bag would be too scary and if she let all the worries
out they might overpower her and her family. Fortunately, a kind
elderly neighbour who's been watching her struggle offers the
young girl some help and asks to open the bag and look inside
with her. Together they are able to decide which worries belong
to her and which do not, which could have action attached to
them and be sorted out, which are other people's and which
are ones she has totally made up. And, of course, those worries
that do belong to her, having seen them in the light of day and
shared them, seem much less heavy and scary. The girl is able
to carry what is left and go off and play with a bag that doesn't
miraculously vanish, but no longer stops her living. This is, of
course, a neat story, but the sentiment has therapeutic merit.

Therapists have an incredibly privileged insight into the
paradoxes of human nature. They make weekly journeys to the
greatest depths of human trauma: death, infertility, infidelity
and depression, as well as the seemingly smaller moments of

pain: a crush we might have on another that goes unnoticed or feelings of jealousy and resentment towards a close friend. Therapists acclimatise themselves to these things not just by training and reading books, but by knowing their own nature and confronting the complicated, painful and embarrassing aspects of themselves that are collectively relegated into a murky puddle of shame within our culture. Because of this, we can share anything and everything with our therapist – and they will meet it with curiosity, compassion and care. A good therapist who offers a combination of empathy and challenge, both a gentle hand and a kick up the arse, will always help us to return to a place of balance when we come up against it all.

This is possible, because therapists are, unconditionally, on our side. A therapist should have your back and they are there to help you navigate the things we so often find hard: trusting others, coping with our emotions, communicating effectively, understanding ourselves, honouring our potential and feeling relatively authentic, confident and unashamed. If you really don't feel your therapist is right for you, and have taken that to the conversation, then move on – bad therapy experiences are real, so use your gut instincts.

THINGS YOU SHOULD KNOW ABOUT THERAPY:

» Make sure you select an accredited therapist. Use regulatory bodies like BACP (British Association for Counselling and Psychotherapy) and UKCP (The UK Council for Psychotherapy).

» You don't have to stick with the first therapist you meet. In your first session, you want to experience comfort. You want to feel the therapist has empathy, understanding and the ability to see ahead of you. A first session is not a lifelong commitment. Try not to put lots of pressure on it to go perfectly – or to stick with it if it wasn't a good fit. Shop around.

» Make some time. Virtual sessions are brilliant because they allow you to slip therapy seamlessly into your daily routine, but it's really important that you allow yourself some time before and after the session to sit with your feelings and digest them before diving into your next task.

» Sometimes you're not going to like or enjoy therapy. It can be like going to the gym in that, more often than not, 'having gone' feels a lot better than the actual 'going'.

» You won't have a cinematic breakthrough in every session. It is slower than we all hope it to be; huge epiphanies are rare and don't happen as much as we see on the telly.

» It's OK to write down what you want to talk about. Fifty minutes can be over in a flash. Spontaneity in the therapy room is incredibly important, but when you're already feeling nervous and unsure of what to say in your early sessions, it's OK to have a list of things you want to cover.

» Ask questions. It's OK to be curious. It's OK to question what your therapist is telling you. Therapy is a two-way street and it shouldn't feel like you've taken the backseat in your sessions.

» Know that coaching and therapy are not the same. Coaching looks at the future, setting goals and thinking about things more practically. It is widely unmoderated as a profession and, unless stated, coaches do not have therapy experience.

» We don't need to know the exact reason we are going to therapy. We can just arrive exactly as we are.

» Try not to pretend, lie or make things up. Practise saying what you are thinking and feeling. It's your time; use it to your advantage. The person that gains from truthfulness is you.

» Level the playing field. You know yourself best – the therapist is there to guide, support and challenge. If something doesn't feel right or helpful, call it out. (We spoke with someone once who'd had nine months of therapy with an elderly therapist who had slept through most of their 50-minute sessions and they had not said anything, believing it was part of the process that they didn't understand!)

» If you do decide to leave therapy after a number of sessions, it's useful for you if you make that clear to the therapist, so you can discuss and plan the ending. This bodes well for future endings in your life and gives you the opportunity to fully explore the ending, making it theoretically useful for you.

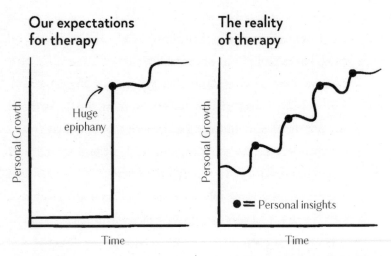

What therapy is really like

Therapy is not the be-all and end-all solution to your happiness. It isn't the golden ticket to never feeling crap again in life. But it is a really important ritual in the toolbox you can begin to build up for yourself. It can be something you engage with once for a period of time or that you return to at different stages in your life. It is a dedicated space that is focused on your self-exploration and this is a key component to being able to grow through what you go through.

WHEN THERAPY DOESN'T FEEL POSSIBLE

We know that therapy might not feel like an option for you – sometimes the cost is too high, sometimes we can struggle to find the right therapist, sometimes we feel we can't face it or have nowhere to begin. Therapy does not have to be the oracle of change (it is, of course, really helpful if and when it becomes possible for you). When it isn't, things to consider include:

» **Find a safe place.** Can you identify a place you feel safest, nurtured and yourself? This might be walking in nature, being in bed or snuggled in a cosy nook in a cafe. Take yourself there when you are struggling and try to just be.

» **Who is your 'old lady'?** Like in the story of the little girl (see page 162), is there a person who you respect, value the opinion of and who can make time and space for you to speak and be listened to? They might help you sort things out, talk things through with you. They might watch as you cry, sit and drink tea with you. They might just be in the same space as you. Understanding who that person or people are can be really helpful for you. Feed back to them about what you find valuable so they understand their worth to you.

» **The bag of worries activity.** Make your own version of the bag of worries experience (see page 162). Write down the key challenges you face – it might be people, places, problems – and try to physically put the bits of paper into groups or even in small pots. What do you have control over and what don't you have control over? What belongs to you really?

These are just some of our ideas, and those of our clients, for ongoing mental maintenance; there are no doubt many more. If you were writing this chapter or telling a friend, what would be your top-priority routines and rituals for mental maintenance?

In the next chapter we'll look at how you can replenish so that you can maintain the strength you need to do this important work.

Chapter 8

Replenish

If you are beginning to do to the work – doing hard things to promote your own growth – know that this deep work can be exhausting. You might feel depleted from the internal action that is beginning. You must replenish yourself in order to have the opportunity for greater success. This simple act of self-love – understanding and acting on the fact you are worth replenishing – can have a significant, positive impact on how you value yourself and on how you grow.

'We cannot pour from an empty cup' is a sentiment often shared for a reason. It's just not possible to magic what is not there. We believe you deserve and should tend to yourself like a piece of fine art, putting care into what it needs to keep its beauty.

Make Space for Joy (and Loveliness)

Joy is an important commodity to keep you replenished. Joy is not to be confused with 'happiness' – we have a preoccupation with wanting or trying to be happy, wondering if everyone else is happy more often than we are or questioning why we aren't happy.

In our experience, feelings of happiness are fleeting and magical but often transient. Joy is more consistent and is cultivated internally. It comes when you make peace with who you are, why you are, and how you are. Happiness tends to be externally triggered and is based on other people, things, places, thoughts and events. Happiness is less predictable and less under our control. Somewhere along the line, we've been sold an unrealistic idea of how happy we should feel in certain situations or in response to particular things, which is why we often feel we are falling short or doing something wrong when we don't feel that happy much of the time.

Joy only appears when we invite and allow it in.

WHAT CAN STOP US EXPERIENCING JOY?

Did you know that a group of ladybirds is called a loveliness? I (Jodie) didn't, but I can remember when I was told it. I was in a group of people and everyone seemed to find this fact really lovely (which I can now relate to). However, at the time, I had no space to find any meaning in what I was hearing and it only served to derail me from my own inner narrative. I remember seeing people's faces and wondering why they seemed so joyful; I thought it kind of stupid, and detached myself from the experience of shared joy. I didn't have the time, space or interest in joy and frivolity. Or so I told myself. It was only some years later when I read something about ladybirds on a nature trail, that I was able to reflect on how elusive the experience of joy was for me at that time. I was so focused on keeping order for myself – ordered thinking, ordered behaviour – that I did not realise how avoidant or unobtainable joy was for me in its frenetic unpredictable nature. How the idea of feeling joyous, of being engaged in something so frivolous, so without purpose other than the very fleeting moment, seemed so irrelevant and banal. I thought I was choosing to rise above such nonsense, but actually, it wasn't a choice at all – I felt I could only stay safe if I denied myself the opportunity to feel joy.

JOY BLOCKERS

Joy and feeling joyous can be inhibited by a number of things. Any of these can mean there will be no space for more replenishing emotions:

» Life events/grief/job struggles/money worries.
» Dissatisfaction in where you are at in life, comparing yourself to others.
» Challenges in relationships being untended to.
» Past trauma or challenges being untended to.
» Being disconnected from yourself/being inauthentic.
» Being tightly wound or stressed.
» Focus on addictions or dependencies.
» Being preoccupied with worry/anxiety/fear.

HOW TO CULTIVATE JOY

There are so many potential opportunities to experience joy if we are able to make space for it. Welcome it in and feel deserving of it – even when you feel at your most rubbish, joy flashes are still possible.

1. Quieten your mind

It's important to be able to tap into your heart rather than your head, your intuition rather than your thinking mind. This clears the way for being able to connect with what sparks joy in you.

2. Find ways to be of service

We know that doing things for others on our terms feels good. We know that when people eat food we have made, see images we create or share smiles, we mostly have a sense of feeling fuller. Find ways that you can be in service to others (without it costing too much, pushing on your boundaries or turning into people-pleasing) and notice if that brings you feelings of joy. Ask for feedback where it is possible so that you can know what impact you are making and use this to store in your joy bank.

3. Find your cheerleading team

We all need a cheerleading squad (or a cheerleader) – people or things that buoy us up and champion our successes, that inspire and motivate us. This might a combination of people, social media accounts that make you feel good, groups of people you share with, or it might be an internalised voice of someone who can be your cheerleader when you need one – maybe someone from your past who had a positive impact. Spend some time thinking about the people in your life who you feel championed by. Identify what it is that they do that makes you feel good and supported, and encourage/invite more of that in.

JOURNAL PROMPT

You might want to create your own internal cheerleader or mascot – make it, draw it, write it:

»   What do they look like?

»   Name them.

»   What do they say, how do they speak?

»   How do you reach or connect to them?

Actively participate with your joy team that supports the fact that you deserve lovely things and you are able to and deserve to welcome joy without combusting. There does not need to be an outcome or purpose to it other than to remember the loveliness, your loveliness and the loveliness of others, and know that we all need to be powered up sometimes.

Champion Community

We are tribal creatures by nature, however modern we may think we are! Being part of a tribe, from an anthropological perspective, means survival. We once relied on a whole community of close-knit people to support our basic needs, from food to childcare. Wherever we are from in the world, we come from an ancestral line that relies heavily on the love, support, knowledge, strength and wisdom of a community.

Communities practised common ownership – they shared things, they protected each other (often from the other tribe down the road). It meant really having each other's back, which felt good and kept people safe. It's why we try to retain such a close bond with our family. It's why we support our football team. It's why we play team sports. We like the vibe of the tribe. We have already explored in this book how vital intimacy, meaningful connection, sharing with others and feeling able to remove our masks is for our well-being. We need to be supported and we also need to support others – it's how we feel able to move past our defences and be more authentic. Being and feeling part of community helps us to grow.

Developed over millions of years of evolution, our instincts make us crave a tribal society. That instinct is a fundamental part of our social fabric, but community spirit and feel is much, much less evident in the world now. We have grown away from the dependency we once had on a direct community and, in that, something has been lost. We have built our existence away from, not towards, each other. The world can feel very non-community even though most of us live within one. This is universal; as technology has grown, community has changed and been reshaped, it lacks the meaning it once had. We can lose the positive impact of community on our well-being unless we cultivate it.

Community exists, but not in the same way. We are missing the authenticity of the community where we could not hide behind an email, a like, a comment. We used to be so intimately in each other's lives that when love was offered it felt real and genuine. We had intimate connections based on much more unfiltered versions of ourselves. We were able to connect more deeply and more frequently, which was good for our mental health. Today, while we are seemingly less reliant on each other in many ways, it does not mean we need each other less. The move away from the fundamental need to trust in others for our survival gives us the licence to be less connected. Modern society is the antithesis to connection. It is highly individualistic. We lack social accountability, have no security from those around us, are constantly surrounded by strangers, and there is a fundamental lack of trust that dangerously undermines the social fabric of society.

This doesn't mean we need to be depended on; we just need to find other ways of experiencing and creating community. We have to work very much harder now to recreate this experience and the many benefits associated with it.

HOW TO BUILD A SENSE OF COMMUNITY

What do you have that you can offer the community that can be given without resentment? How and where can you offer it?

» What is happening in the local community that you might feel OK about getting involved in (jumble trail, cake bakes, local school or community centres, music events)?
» Can you volunteer somewhere that captures your interest?
» Can you start a community initiative that feels creative?

> » Are there wider, virtual communities you can be a part of?
> » Celebrate together: share food, carol sing, arrange a street party.
> » Skill swap.
> » Arrange meet-ups (running, knitting or walking groups).

Refuel and Replenish

Try to make space to understand what fills your cup and build this into your day or week. This might include travel, new adventures, writing, art, looking at insects, running. Is it five minutes in the sun, an eyebrow tint, a dog walk, a cold drink enjoyed in solitude or a coffee with a good friend? Is it a moment to read a book, to cook food for yourself, listen to or play music, dancing, art, stamp collecting? What matters to you?

You will not get all your needs met from one place. Know this! Perhaps you get replenished in areas like family, friends, relationships, work, creativity, hobbies, the arts, play, education, food, social, travel . . . think about how much time you allocate to each and the amount you gain from it. You might need to rebalance how much time and energy you put in one place so that your return is what you need to feel your better self. If you spend a lot of time and energy on something but get little emotional reward, it might need rethinking.

It is useful sometimes to find a metaphor for how and where you get your needs met – a 'replenish station'. We have

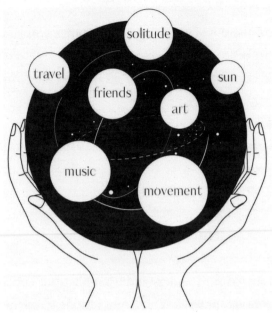

Replenishing stations

a client who thinks of replenishing places as her own private high street of shops, full of things she might need and want. We have another client who has a house with different rooms for different things that he can visit.

Try imagining yourself as an astronaut who has many useful planets in your galaxy you can visit to fuel up, find meaning, to gather useful things you might need to replenish. On a piece of paper, draw yourself with all the refill places that you need/ want in your life and what they provide.

Hold On Tightly, Let Go Lightly

It feels fitting that we bring this chapter to a close with this concept. Hold on to what works for you, what fills you up, what's worth your energy, and let go (sometimes with work) of anything that does not. Let go with conscious grace where you can. But let go. Do not hold on to what doesn't serve you.

Holding on tightly and letting go lightly might look like:

» Understanding your own pain at your kids starting school, but not getting in their way. Hold on to yourself compassionately – 'This is horrid. What do I need?' – but you let go knowing you both need room to grow.

» Knowing that you can hold on tight to relationships, fight for them, work at them, but when you need to, the biggest gain for yourself might be to let go.

» You can hold on to control until it serves you no longer and is restricting you, and then you can let go and empower someone else so that they can do it better.

» You can hold on to your independence, but know that letting others in can be a supportive way of letting go.

Know that when we loosen our grip on things, there is room for us to experience what stays and what goes – we allow the opportunity for choice. We can be reassured, surprised, frightened by what this might uncover, but when we hold on too tight, we are not rewarded in the same way as if we let go and it comes back. Like a dog, or a child, or a returning lover, when they return through choice its feels so much more meaningful.

Even after you do *all* of this you might still feel horrible sometimes because you are human. My (Jodie) son said to me once, during a particularly difficult time, that he didn't have the words to describe exactly how he was feeling, but that he thought he was lost, 'lost somewhere I think I recognise, but it doesn't seem to make sense'. I thought it was a perfect description of an emotional space we often find ourselves in. Uncertain, confused, at odds with ourselves and often quite lost, but somehow it's familiar like we know this place. We can panic at this feeling, desperately grasp to what holds us in an anchored space, often unhelpfully anchoring to the things that support us to resist change. But it's at times like these that it might be useful to refer to the tips in this chapter. To be reassured that here, within these maintenance ideas, there might be a place where you can find some support.

Sometimes we just need to know we are in a shit place and be compassionate with ourselves, rather than always pushing for change, which can be exhausting. You are not a never-ending self-improvement project – we don't need to be constantly improving and toiling on ourselves otherwise we'll combust.

Sometimes we might be at peace – let's just accept that for a second rather than looking for the next change phase. Let yourself rest from your self-work sometimes. Let yourself off the hook and remind yourself that you are enough just as you are.

In the next section we'll be exploring change and some bigger issues that might need more untangling. Keep a tight hold of the maintenance tips we've covered so far – they will give you a good, solid base to grow from.

PART 3

The Knife-Edge of Change

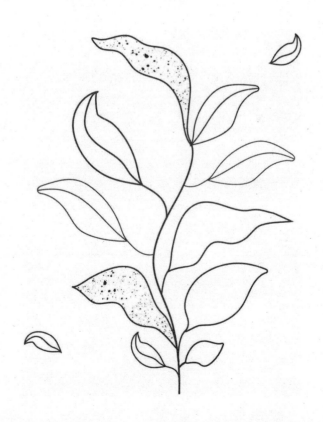

We often find clients come to see us in the pain that comes before the change. They have an idea that change would be helpful to their growth, but they cannot get there alone. They don't often fully know that's why they've arrived – they'll mostly say they don't feel great, their confidence is struggling, their anxiety is high, they're not sleeping – but as their story unfolds, there will almost always be an element of change emerging or that needs to emerge.

Whether that is leaving a relationship, changing the shape of a relationship, becoming a parent, changing career, changing their own relationship to life, when we get stuck before the leap, it can feel exhausting and depleting. When we sit on the precipice of change, we often find ourselves on a metaphorical knife-edge – on the blade – which is really uncomfortable and energy-sapping. Indecision, uncertainty, weighing up pros and cons, and desperation to mitigate the inevitable grief and uncertainty that often accompanies change is tiring.

You might find that you ruminate in this place, look for guarantees, make lists of what might or might not happen – one day you're going to do it, the next day you can't even think about it. You get stuck in the elevator going from one position to the next. This is inevitable – we are human and we want to spare ourselves the pain, yet we experience worse by staying put.

We can find ourselves on this knife-edge for long and exhausting periods. Perhaps you have periods of apathy, feeling grey, lacklustre, where you can't consider the idea or get involved in making change. Things feel perhaps a bit hopeless. Even uncomfortably, we settle into this space, and though this can sometimes bring peace, it can also contribute to a setting in of not feeling good enough, of not honouring our potential, of not feeling ourselves, or of resentment, rage and just generally feeling a bit shitty.

We all at some point have to move off the knife-edge in order for growth to happen. In this section, we are going to share some of the practices and actions you can take to invite change in. If you do not normally practise the suggestions that follow, this is an opportunity to try to do things differently to bring about change. They might offer you the impetus to move from this knife-edge. Leaning into these can help you make the jump that might support you to move forward. They can help you alter life subtly and significantly.

The encouragement from us in this section is that when the change is internal for you, it can impact the outside parts of your life for the better. Mind shifts and taking regular action can bring change that you might never imagine.

Chapter 9

Dealing With Change

Humans really are the most capable, resourceful and resilient creatures that have ever lived on earth. History has shown that when change comes to humanity – either on the global level or on a personal level – we are generally pretty good at it. We are good at adapting. Yet, despite this, we often refuse to embrace change.

Most people will tell you that they find change difficult. This is because change can mean things falling apart and also new beginnings, which makes it exciting, thrilling and creative and at other times full of dread, sadness and confusion. For this reason, we usually meet change with anxiety and resistance, mainly because change is uncomfortable, unsettling and full of uncertainty. Uncertainty kindles fear and often a fear of failure, which is incredibly hard for us to bear – so most of us choose to be unhappy rather than uncertain. This can be found in the story of someone being in a marriage for ten years longer than they wanted to, but choosing to stay because of paralysing fear: fear of being seen as a failure for ending the marriage, fear of having to go on dates to find a new partner and the possibility of being rejected, and fear of being single and alone. Or the person who chooses to stay in a job that makes them miserable and leaves them feeling unsatisfied because they fear not getting a new one.

Our brains have evolved to find peace and comfort in familiarity, so fear of change is natural and instinctive. As a result, so many of us try our hardest to avoid change, but it inevitably catches up with us. As therapists, we are kind of in the business of change and, in our years of practice, we have come to learn that sometimes we choose change and *sometimes change chooses us*. Regardless of how much we fear it because outcomes are unknown, change runs alongside the timelines of our lives at a steady pace and, every so often, it elbows its way in, shifting our trajectory. Sometimes it wakes us up in the dead of night. Sometimes it greets us when the sun comes up. Sometimes it reaches us through an unexpected phone call or text. Sometimes it comes into our lives ferociously like a storm and clears a path for us. Sometimes we sigh into it, exhausted and unable to go on with our lives in the same way. Sometimes we are propelled into change by beautiful surprises, moments of luminosity or horrifying traumas. Sometimes change may simply come after getting sick of our own bullshit.

Change and Transition

In our race through changes, our attention can easily fixate on the change itself, and we spend much less time on processing transition. The two words are commonly used interchangeably, but they are different. Change is external, organisational, quicker,

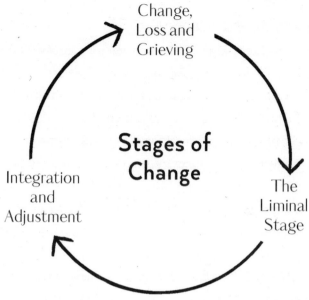

Change,
Loss and
Grieving

**Stages of
Change**

Integration
and
Adjustment

The
Liminal
Stage

Stages of change

more visible, more predictable, physical and tangible. Transition is internal, personal, slower, less visible, less predictable, psychological and intangible. Change is something that happens to us, whether we choose it or it chooses us. Transition, on the other hand, is something that we ourselves *have* to go through. It's what occurs within us (psychologically, emotionally) as we go through change. Change can happen quite fast, while transition usually happens more slowly.

When it comes to navigating change, it serves us to attend to the transition(s) that flows from it. Look at any theoretical model within transition psychology and it will generally point to three phases that we move through when faced with change; they read as linear, but they are more cyclical, and each of us will experience them in our own unique way:

1. CHANGE, LOSS AND GRIEVING

We enter this initial stage of transition when we are first confronted with change. This stage is usually marked with resistance and big emotions (fear, denial, anger, sadness, disorientation) because we are being challenged to let go of something that, more often than not, brings us comfort, familiarity, affirmation, meaning or connection. We can meet this stage during big life moments like leaving/starting a job, moving to a new place, getting a promotion, the death of a loved one, becoming a parent, having a miscarriage, getting divorced or separating, turning 30, 40, 50 and so on.

Whether it is a positive change or a challenging one, regularly accompanying change are its close friends 'grief' and 'loss'. Grief is experienced during death but also in other losses, the kind that psychotherapist Julia Samuel coined 'living losses': lost routines, lost connections, lost habits and habitats, loss of family structures, loss of assumptions that everything will be OK, lost jobs and career progression, loss of feelings of freedom before becoming a parent and so on. Whenever a change occurs, even for the better, there is the potential for experiences of grief and loss. Sometimes, we must grieve what we are letting go of, or leaving behind, before we can start taking steps forward to growth. This process can be painful – so painful that it might feel easier to stay where we are comfortable rather than go where we can flourish.

We easily mistake grief for a sign that we are doing the wrong thing, but we have to remember that grief is a natural part of the process of change. When we allow grief to be valid instead of something to overlook or dismiss, we can continue on our path, even with the grief that might come along with it. Embracing the grief of change is challenging, but the more we can let ourselves experience it fully, the lighter the load is as we move ahead in our lives.

2. THE LIMINAL STAGE
(THE UNCOMFORTABLE IN-BETWEEN)

Liminality (an anthropological term meaning 'threshold') describes a sense of ambiguity or disorientation that happens in the middle stage of a rite of passage. Suppose we were to think about significant periods of change as rites of passage, this liminal stage is the point at which we are no longer who we were before the change happened, and we are not quite who we will be when it is completed. At this stage, we stand at the threshold between the old way of structuring our identity, community, personal and interpersonal worlds, and a new way.

Let's look at some of those big life moments and what the liminal stage might look like: becoming a parent and finding yourself struggling over the loss of your identity as a professional, a partner, a person free to travel spontaneously, and your new identity as a parent, responsible for the life of a small human for the rest of your life. When getting divorced, you might find yourself holding the tension between your old identity – which was wrapped up in your partner and family and that gave you a sense of belonging and purpose – and your new identity, which can feel emergent, lonely, liberating or exciting. When moving to a new place, you might find yourself torn between two geographical locations: an old place that was familiar and gave you a sense of locality, and a new place, and trying to adjust, find a sense of grounding and build a sense of community.

In this liminal stage, we are often confused, uncertain and impatient. We are holding the tension between the old and the new. We might be feeling resentful towards the change, have low moods, ambivalence and anxiety, while questioning our identity. We experience resistance to the change and, like all seasons of growth, it is probable we are going to lose something: we lose familiarity and the comfort we find there, we lose the things we hold on to, to keep us safe.

Picture it a bit like being on a beach. We are not entirely out at sea, wading in the deep and completely unknown of the water, but nor are we inland, and our feet are not planted firmly on solid, certain ground. Like the beach, anything can wash up. Waves of emotion move in and out, sometimes gently, sometimes smashing us against the rocks.

We might find ourselves lingering here for days, weeks and months, falling in and out of periods of overthinking. In seasons of change, none of us knows what will happen next, but this doesn't stop any of us overthinking and trying to conjure up what might be. Here, all we are doing is trying to control the future, and when we're trying to control the future we're not thinking about the now – and that can cause so much anxiety and worry. It stops us from being able to integrate and adjust.

When you are in this liminal stage, your emotional unrest usually comes from your disconnectedness from the present.

You might become pulled into the future, catastrophising over what it will bring, forgetting to be in the present and observe what's happening around you. In these moments, it serves us to reflect on what's happening.

JOURNAL PROMPT

Grab your journal and, thinking about a change that might be happening for you or a situation that you might be in, respond to each of these questions:

» What has happened?

» What past events led up to this?

» How were you involved in the development of this situation?

» How were others involved in the development of this situation?

» What part of this situation do you have control over?

» What part of this situation do you *not* have control over?

» How are you responding or reacting to this situation?

» How is your own response making you feel? Are you judging your feelings harshly? Are you 'should-ing' yourself? (When we 'should' ourselves it can become persecutory and is not very productive. If you're saying to yourself 'I should', what happens if you change that to 'I could'? The latter can be more empowering.)

Finally, look at it, name it and think about how you can objectively look at the situation. You can use a simple structure:

Stressful reality	Ways to objectively accept reality
I've left my job and I have no income next month.	It's OK to worry about money; I've just left my job. If I apply for jobs I can earn money, pay my bills and have money. I am going to update my CV, apply to jobs and ask someone to help me in doing so.
I've moved to a new place and I feel lonely.	Of course I'll feel lonely sometimes – I've just left somewhere familiar and I'm in a new place. I'm going to think about what communities I can connect with here. I'm going to look for Meetups, groups or workshops with people that share my interests. I will form connections with my local coffee shop through daily interactions. I can do this and still call and connect with people in my life who I used to see regularly.

Bring yourself back to the present

Periods of change, or distressing situations, can cause us to obsess about the future or our fate. But your anchor is this moment – you can return to it to find peace, simply by remembering to be here in the present. This prevents you from getting too lost in anxious thought. Here you can remind yourself to stick with the situation at hand: 'Why is this so unbearable? Why should I be fearful right now?'

Maybe you have a hot drink close by, maybe you're in the company of a loved one. Or maybe you're uncomfortable, stressed or struggling. Wherever you find yourself, when you separate your current experience at this moment from your thoughts, is it as overwhelming or terrifying as you expect? Or is your mind elsewhere – somewhere that is far worse, that doesn't exist?

You can support this process by getting in touch with your body and paying attention to how it's responding to change and the stress it brings. Short-term strategies start in the body; a ritual involving breathing will help you relax and restore, so here is one to try:

BREATHE AND RELAX
Anchor now. Breathe deeply ten times from your belly. Feel your feet on the ground.

1. Get yourself into a relaxed, comfortable position. You could be sitting on a chair or on the floor, on a yoga mat or a cushion. Try to keep your back upright, but not strained. Rest your hands wherever they're comfortable. Relax your jaw.
2. Bring your attention to your body and invite your body to relax. Turn your attention to the sensations you are experiencing – the touch, the connection with the chair or the floor. Do your best to relax any tight areas of tension. Breathe. Drop your shoulders.
3. Tune into the rhythm of your breath. The gentle rise and fall. Feel the flow of it, breathe in and out. Notice where you feel your breath in your body. It might be in your belly, it may be in your chest or throat or

in your nostrils. See if you can feel the sensations of breath, one breath at a time. Notice the pauses in between each breath.

4. As you do this, no doubt your mind will start to wander. You may start thinking about other things. If this happens, it is not a problem. Try to notice that your mind has moved away from your body, and as you breathe, gently redirect your attention right back to the breathing. You can come back with a centring word: it might be 'breath', or 'body', or whatever else works for you.

5. Stay here for five to seven minutes. Notice your breath, in silence. From time to time, you'll get lost in thought, then return to your breath and your body.

6. After a few minutes, once again notice your body, your whole body, seated here. Notice your body from the inside. Let yourself relax even more deeply and then thank yourself for this moment.

From this place of calm, we are in a much stronger position to support our whole selves to allow total acceptance of 'this moment' or of 'this reality at this moment'. Sometimes it's too easy to become fixated on events or situations over which you have no power or control. But rather than focusing on moving the unmovable, you can set your sights on what you can control.

TIME FOR REFLECTION

Ask yourself:

»   What, today, can I be in control of?

»   What is within my reach?

»   What might I need to commit to accepting?

Practise radical acceptance

When we are faced with a change, we often fight reality. Recognise when you're doing this: you might be feeling resentful, thinking your life shouldn't be this way, thinking if only X changed, you would be happy. When you accept change, you give permission for change to happen. The uncomfortable feelings that come along with change cannot overstay their welcome. It's important you do this without judgement. In other words, we do not choose parts of reality to accept and parts to reject. In this place of grounding, you are able to better evaluate your level of control.

This is a challenging, exhausting stage, but if you can bear it long enough, it can be a space of creativity, innovation and renewal as you map new ways of being.

3. INTEGRATION AND ADJUSTMENT

In this stage we move towards deeper acceptance. Life is not the same, and nor will it be again. We still move in and out of sadness and grieving, but we begin to have more energy and become open to new experiences. We carry with us what we have lost, but we also grow around the losses we have experienced. We begin to find resolve. Grief becomes unfrozen. We find meaning, reconstruct our identity, adjust our expectations, rediscover hope and revise our attachment to the thing or person we have lost within the change that has happened. We begin to calibrate.

Most of us want to skip straight to this stage, but we can remain stuck if we are unwilling to experience the uncomfortable parts of growth and transition first. We won't move forward or grow if we avoid the task. Remaining stuck and comfortable is far less rewarding than trudging forward through the mud and emerging a stronger, wiser, braver, whole version of ourselves.

Damon (36) came to see me (Jodie) for support with 'stress' symptoms, foremost a persistent skin condition that caused sore, itchy skin. We worked together over three years. Damon seemed on the surface to manage his everyday life well – he didn't locate feeling stressed about the relationships he had with people, and his work and private life were in what appeared to be good-enough shape. When I asked him what he felt stressed about, he said he wasn't sure.

We worked a little on his family history and we identified that his skin symptoms began when he was 19 and his mother died. I wasn't immediately able to identify his fear of change until the first Christmas of our work together. We were speaking about Christmas decorations and he said he didn't have the stress of decorating as he used his mother's artificial tree every year (she had died on New Year's Day).

I asked him about possibly buying a new tree this year and how that would feel. He immediately began scratching his skin quite frantically. From here we were able to begin to see the patterns in his fear around change, in small details of his life: his mother's shopping bag with one handle that he continued to use, the aftershave she bought him, the same bed linen.

These tributes can sometimes help us feel closer to those we've lost, but, in Damon's case, they were acting as a prison for both his grief emotions and his growth. We incrementally began to discuss, honour and let go of some of the things he was holding on to, which was both upsetting and destabilising for him, but ultimately freeing. His skin condition became much less severe and he began to celebrate and look forward to the marking of old rituals and the introduction of change. Each one he said 'felt like a step forward'. Here we see that dealing with, and living through, the change can be painful, but the avoidance of it can keep us very stuck.

Inviting Change

Change is inevitable, regardless of whether you choose it or not. We are in a constant state of change – our bodies, our minds, our processes. We were built to change and adapt, and in the most part we are good at it (that doesn't always make it comfortable; in fact it's most often uncomfortable). We see it in our bodies, the way we grow upwards, outwards, in weird ways! The same applies to our lives – we outgrow our clothes, habits, people, jobs, houses, roles . . . you will, in fact, be growing and changing even as you read these pages. Even so, change is almost always destabilising, even just momentarily, even when we are welcoming and embracing it. When we are ready and prepared for change, we will always have to move through a period of letting something go in order to make space for something else, which can be both liberating and fear-inducing.

Sometimes we are ready for change, but we wait too long. Sometimes we don't jump at all and get so wedded to where we are that change can feel impossible – we get stuck. Sometimes we move too quickly without consideration, and then run into challenges. Sometimes, like the ending of relationships, redundancy, or illness or death, change comes for us and pushes us off-kilter – we don't happen to it, it happens to us.

TIME FOR REFLECTION

How do you feel about change?

- » What significant/impactful changes have you made?
- » What was the period before the change like?
- » What did it feel like after?
- » What changes didn't you/haven't you made?
- » How do you feel about those changes?
- » How did change exist or not exist in your family?
- » Is there anything you'd like to change in your life right now?
- » What, if anything, feels possible about it?
- » What feels less possible?
- » How does that make you feel?

Ask yourself once, and then again, and see if your answers are the same.

ACCEPT WHAT NEEDS CHANGING

The first challenge you might face is accepting that change is needed. Carl Jung said, 'we cannot change anything until we accept it'. This can involve the horrid element of taking a long, hard look in the mirror and facing what we don't want to see about ourselves. You might feel this after the third night out drinking when you wake up feeling crapper than crap, or after another hopeless meeting with your boss when you're all out of options for making it better. Perhaps you pack the kids off to school in another screaming fit that makes you feel rubbish, or can't face retuning to your flat share. Maybe you look in the mirror and hate your hair, or sit in traffic and really wonder what you are doing, or you roll away from your partner in bed and feel too alone for it to bearable any longer.

Whatever motivates you to really consider change, in order to make it possible you will need to face yourself in the equation. Often this can be shame-inducing and momentarily quite yucky. Whatever it is that prompts you, know that change – and therefore growth – is possible.

PRACTISE LITTLE AND OFTEN

Don't try to change everything at once. Practise little and often, for example, changing up where you get your coffee, leaving work on time, going home instead of to the pub, changing your brand of trainers or what you cook for tea. Prove to yourself your adaptability: say no when you would normally say yes. Show yourself that you can make changes, and survive, so that implicitly you have a sense that change is possible.

When you come to face much bigger changes and begin to make them, that is the time to keep other things more stable. For example, in the midst of a separation, your local coffee shop might feel reassuring. In the time of moving house you might find comfort in the same bedcover or candle scent. Treat yourself gently and with compassion, but with the belief that you can change.

MAKE THE UNSAID SAID

Holding on to unspoken truths can manifest in our bodies. It can dominate our waking and sleeping thoughts and impact our general sense of well-being. When we leave our truth unsaid, we deny our own reality. This is a communication to ourselves that what we think/feel does not matter enough to give it space. Avoidance or denial just compounds our emotions and can contribute to feelings of isolation and distress. No one really relishes uncomfortable conversations and most of us will do anything to avoid potential conflict, often allowing things to build until they are consuming. We stack the emotional stakes high in conversations that might be triggering or challenging for us. We might be terrified of how the other person feels or might respond to what we are saying; we may fear causing upset or anger. Having established a relationship that is built on some precarious untruths, we might be afraid of exposing our vulnerabilities or holding a boundary.

The conversation that needs to be had will suck your attention and energy until you actually have it. Having these difficult conversations is really vital to our growth and brings immediate feelings of relief; when we let down our guard and are able to soften and hear others more, we are able to connect authentically.

HOW TO APPROACH EMOTIONALLY CHARGED CONVERSATIONS

First think why this conversation matters to you. Why is it charged? Work out what you are feeling before you go any further.

1. Think about what you would like the outcome to be and why. What if you let go of the idea of a definitive outcome? Enquire further than the pay rise, or the custody outcome, or the party you weren't invited to. Search a little further and ask what it is you really need from the conversation. Perhaps you need to feel valued, cared for, seen, heard, understood, included? Use this information to lean in more softly.

2. Practise beforehand, with a friend or in prayer, so that the words have airtime and you play around with how you feel and what you say.

3. Begin sentences with 'I' not 'you'. Start with how you feel, not what they have or haven't done. It's very difficult to argue about someone's feelings. It also immediately connects others to your human side if you start with 'I feel . . .'.

4. Tease out the space in the conversation for exploration and understanding, rather than jumping to an exit. The bigger gain for you might be the experience and meaning rather than the outcome you imagine.

BE OPEN TO INTIMACY

Intimacy is a game changer in terms of change. When we are able to generate more intimacy within our relationships, we have the opportunity for deeper connection, support, problem-sharing and solving. Intimacy can give us a sense of security or power and of self-actualisation, which all make change more possible – both self-generated and imposed change. We can build our flexibility and adaptability when we experience more intimacy in our lives and this powers us up and enables us to grow.

Firstly know this: intimacy is not just sex! There are four types of intimacy:

1. Emotional intimacy: Mutual sharing of feelings, deep communication, disclosing your inside self, the things in your

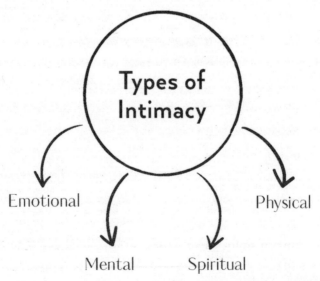

Types of intimacy

head and heart, sharing things which might feel difficult, upsetting, confusing and shameful. In emotional intimacy, we expose our true selves.

How: Try to have more meaningful conversations with people you trust. Share how you're feeling or what's going on for you, even if it isn't neat and tidy. Share things that are not working out, the challenges and the struggles. Tell them you are feeling alone if you are. Encourage a sense of non-judgement between the two of you that validates and welcomes honesty.

Watch outs: Fake intimacy, telling stories about yourself you feel disconnected to in order to control or direct a response from the listener, dramatising events/your experience in order to make it feel more valid, making things up about yourself or others to create a false sense of intimacy. For example, saying things like 'Oh yes that happened to me', even if it didn't. Intoxication and over-sharing when you really need intimacy can create experiences that aren't emotionally safe.

2. Mental intimacy: Meeting of minds: it feels satisfying, challenging and possibly stimulating. Bouncing ideas off each other, meeting your intellectual match or feeling creatively or intellectually inspired when you are together. You might share professional experiences, you might be planning a business opportunity together, or really value each other's opinions around work, the arts, like the same things, or disagree passionately. It might include some healthy competition. Championing, and feeling a little inspired by each other.

How: Share work challenges or career confusion, ask for support and advice when you need it. Share the joys and successes and invest in others' journeys. Be a champion for each other.

Watch outs: Notice repeating feelings of jealousy or envy if they emerge. Share those feelings, talk it through and use them to support the intimacy, not destroy it. Avoid fierce competition and stay true to your truths within the relationships. Be inside each other's real journeys rather than outside harbouring difficult feelings.

3. Spiritual intimacy: This might be a set of values or ethics you share, or spiritual practices that you can unite on. It might be anything from yoga to religion. Perhaps you practise together, celebrate common events, and understand each other's views on big life things.

How: Share ideas and experiences. Show each other what speaks to your spirituality and share in joyful things that have an impact on you. It might be a place, a view, a meditation, a piece of music, a poem. Find ways to be expansive in what you share and how you include each other.

Watch outs: Look out for superiority or a desire for excellence in the topic that unites you because this might create a harmful power dynamic and be avoidant of intimacy. Watch out for trying to rescue others or impart your views too strongly or over-challenge particular views.

4. Physical intimacy: Physical intimacy and sexual intimacy are two ways that people show affection for each other. Sex and intimacy aren't always the same thing and we can often confuse them as being so. Sex is a biological function, but physical intimacy is often an indicator of a deeper intimate relationship and can happen with or without sex. We can be involved in very physically intimate relationships which involve truth, compassion, care and a deep understanding of each other, where sex is an important part of developing and building on a sense of intimacy. But we can also have physical intimacy with people we have deep and meaningful relationships with, which do not involve sex. We might find this in families, in close friendships and with people we feel seen by. It might involve hand-holding, hugging, being in close proximity in an uncensored way. Being in each other's company and feeling at ease with each other.

How: In your sexual relationships, if you need something more intimate, talk about what you are hoping for. Find ways to develop intimacy by talking through your fears, hopes and experiences of the relationship as well as your sexual desires. Developing dialogue which is based on truth can deepen your relationship and help you attune.

Watch outs: Mistaking sex for intimacy or looking for intimacy and offering or accepting sex as a way of getting it. This can be an act of desperation and/or exposure of our deepest vulner- abilities. We can confuse sex or someone's desire for sex as a substitute for the intimacy we need. This might cause us further pain when intimacy is not felt. It can also be a defence against intimacy – the very thing you are searching for.

TIME FOR REFLECTION

» What does intimacy mean to you?

» What does intimacy feel like?

» Who do you have intimate relationships with?

NEED FOR CONNECTION

Loneliness isn't just the absence of people, but an absence of meaningful connections in our lives. If you have feelings of loneliness and want to work on this area of your life, here are some suggestions:

» Start small and build up. Make a commitment to spend at least 15 minutes a day with people you love, whether in person, on video or by phone. That time can be valuable in helping boost our mood and can make others feel better, too.

» Quality time is key. For those interactions that you do have, eliminate distractions. Listen deeply, share more openly and model vulnerability. Push yourself to share things that really matter, how you're really doing and voice the unsaid things.

» Lean into community care. Look at ways to serve others. Cook a meal, check on a neighbour or call a friend. Service is powerful because it breaks those harmful cycles by shifting the focus from ourselves to someone else in the context of a positive interaction.

In this chapter we've looked at just a few of the ways that you can invite change into your life, and build your mental wellness and flexibility. Lean in to the challenge of our invitations and return to them when you feel lost.

In the chapters that follow, we'll look at some of the bigger changes people face in life – divorce and separation, grief and loss, and parenthood – and show you ways in which you can navigate through them.

Chapter 10

Divorce and Separation

The ending of a relationship is one of the biggest periods of transition you can go through – the preparing for, when it actually happens and then life after. It is often not given the gravitas it deserves in terms of consideration to our mental health and the huge amount of change involved, both internally and externally, to grow through the experience.

When we begin relationships we can never be certain of the journey they will take. We are taking an emotional risk when we allow others in – sometimes it's easy and sometimes it's not; sometimes it's positive and sometimes it's not. But we always have the potential, whatever the experience, to learn, mostly about ourselves and sometimes about others.

When we enter into a relationship of any type, we bring with us the complexities of our past, our past experiences of relationships and the experiences we have had around love – both loving and being loved. We don't come in as a blank canvas. This will, of course, determine how able we are to take the risk of intimacy, how we attach and how we relate to others.

We know that love in itself is not enough to guarantee a happy ever after – that is a cinematic construct. In reality, relationships are arduous at times, and need care, attention and work from both parties. That doesn't mean they aren't nutritious or good. That's the reality of all relationships. You change and grow. You'll have periods of grief, poor mental health, stress, apathy, low and high moods. You'll go through different life phases and so will your partner or partners, and all of this will have an impact on how you do and don't relate to each other. The ups-and-downs, even the down-downs do not need to mean the relationship is doomed or over.

However, sometimes we are faced with such enormous relational difficulties that staying together hinders our growth. We don't share the same values anymore and sometimes we just fall out of love. In fact, we outgrow each other and this can feel like loss of love (that in itself doesn't need to mean the end, but it can). Just like a good show, we need to know when the end should come, even if it does feel difficult and upsetting. Often we have a sense that we have reached an end, and that is OK. As with any change, even when it's right, it can feel immeasurably hard.

We cannot, even though the bible suggests we should, commit to love the same person forever. Well, not in a way that means we must stay together at all costs. We can do our very best to try to stay in love, if that is what we want and need. We can try to negotiate the challenges and put the work in, work hard on what it means to be together, to be alone together, to negotiate challenges and keep relating. But, as the life expectancy of people increases, the openness to different types of relationships grows and a call to be more authentic resonates across us, we will be faced with the reality of relationships ending or ending relationships.

Marriages do come to a close, and moving apart from partners that you once could not imagine life without may happen. But while endings like this might be deeply uncomfortable, they are vital to our growth. The quality or length of the relationship does not necessarily determine the impact of the ending, and the endings of both healthy and unhealthy relationships bring with them their own joys, sadness, anger and confusion . . . the list of feelings is endless.

You will experience all the endings you have ever had in each new ending you face, so sometimes your response to the present ending brings with it many ghosts from your past. What endings you experience in your childhood, how those were handled and experienced by you, what you witnessed, how you were cared for (or not) through those endings will impact the present.

Navigating the landscape between loving somebody, but knowing that you need to act in accordance with your own needs – even when those needs mean leaving, departing or hurting someone – can be terrible. Making the decision to leave and the aftermath of leaving and being left, all encounter their own challenges. Each and every one of you will pave your own unique course with it.

We hope we can meet you here, as we hope you will meet yourself at the end of anything, with a little compassion, some understanding and some hope for what's to come. However, we hold deep respect for the fact that we have not been inside your relationship and we cannot know for sure if the ending is right or not. We get asked time and time again in the therapy room: 'Should I leave, is it over?' and we always say, 'I can't answer that.' What we *can* do is be here in the voices of hundreds of endings we have weathered with our clients and ourselves. We have both been through relationship endings and heartbreak – we get it, we've lived it, we know how messy and difficult it can be.

Profound emotional turmoil as the result of major life transitions is a 'phase of life issue'. Divorce is one of these and is recognised by the Holmes and Rahe Stress Scale as the 'second most stressful life event a person can experience, second only to the death of a spouse'. During and after splits, you may find yourself isolating yourself from family and friends, experiencing deep insecurity, acting out in destructive and uncharacteristic ways, having intrusive thoughts and feeling an overwhelming sense of hopelessness. It might feel impossible to imagine a hopeful future where your heart is not broken (of course, our hearts do not really 'break', but we do experience profound loss during some endings). You might feel as if the ground has vanished beneath your feet and you cannot get steady. You might feel jubilation or deep relief after prolonged periods of indecision, when making a decision to leave or when things come to an end. You might not have a clue how you're feeling from one minute to the next. It's all really OK.

We see some things over and over when relationships end and wanted to share some of the most common ones here, in the hope that they might offer you some solace when the transition feels at its bleakest.

Dealing with Judgement

We are constantly judging others – this is a fact. We are also constantly being judged. It's just what we do as humans. How we let, or don't let, this impact us is the important thing. You will be particularly open to the impact of judgement (some real and some imagined) when you are feeling vulnerable and small, which might happen during a relationship ending.

Do share that you feel judged and explore whether there is truth in how you feel – be bold, ask questions and try not to shy away from confronting your uncomfortable feelings, even though this might be a time when you feel at your most vulnerable. If you turn inwards, it can build a layer of further hurt and resentment. Leaning in can act as a way of galvanising relationships that might support you and giving distance to those that might not; it lowers the mask and encourages intimacy. Try to give voice to the way you feel judged and get underneath the skin of it. Ask people how the situation makes *them* feel, what's coming up for them, how they are relating to your situation . . . try to tease out what's going on rather than letting the feeling of being judged attack you to the point of withdrawal.

When there is bereavement in our lives, families and friends surround the bereaved, religions have rituals, employers give compassionate leave, therapy is easily suggested and taken. However, divorce or separation is often viewed very differently. Instead of presenting a united front, family and friends typically take sides, religion has a less emphatic view on the topic, and it can all collude to feel shame-inducing. People can be very unfriendly about this topic and take separation deeply personally. Most people find watching or being connected to endings destabilising; it activates their own fears, concerns, shame about themselves and often they project it on to you.

You may find that you do lose a closeness to people you were once close to, and it's important that you try to communicate as best you can and understand when friendships are not friendly anymore. When we say 'friendly', we understand that friendships will have challenges, they will have conflict and that they'll grow and evolve, but if underneath you don't feel valued or respected, it might be time to reconsider how that friendship supports your life.

HOW TO MANAGE CONFLICT IN RELATIONSHIPS

If you're struggling with conflict – within any of your relationships – here are some ways that might make it a bit easier:

» Use 'I' statements. An 'I' statement reflects your feelings, perceptions and experiences. Using the word 'you' during conflict has the opposite effect: it points fingers at the other's feelings, behaviour or personality.

» Focus on one issue. Don't bring up past arguments and keep it to the matter at hand. Don't lay out all of your relationship problems at once. The more problems you try to air, the less likely they are to be solved.

» Protect your partner/friend's triggers. Whether we like it or not, we are affected by the raw spots in others' pasts, just as they are affected by ours. Working around their triggers with compassion can stop conflict from escalating. Don't know them? Ask.

Also know that you are changing and evolving, and some relationships cannot evolve with you. Just because your decision to move on in a relationship might not suit everyone's views, it doesn't mean you need to be treated without love and compassion.

It's also important to get into contact with how you are judging yourself. Sometimes it is harsh, sometimes it is valid, sometimes it is damaging; sometimes it'll be old habits or learnt behaviour which serve you no purpose in more contentment or growth.

WAYS TO DEAL WITH FEELINGS OF BEING JUDGED

Often, when judgements impact you, there is a seed of truth or merit in what we feel, even though it can be really uncomfortable. Judging in life is inevitable, both by ourselves and others. What's useful is to work out what can you take – if anything – from it to deepen your understanding about yourself and what you can let go of.

» The first thing to do is to see if you can locate what is resonating – can you accept yourself within it as being imperfect? For example, 'everyone thinks I'm disloyal for leaving': while this may not be true, what might be more realistic is that you have disappointed the expectations of others, and say, broken a marriage vow, which might upset some people.

» Ask how you feel about *yourself* within this situation: are you judging yourself? Are you feeling uncomfortable with how you have behaved? If so, what does your inner critic tell you about that? Are you hearing this reflected by others? What can you learn from your discomfort?

» Can you do anything to make things feel better for yourself? This might include an explanation, connecting with those feeling disconnected, sharing your truth, saying sorry.

» Whose voice do you hear in the judgement? Can you reframe it to sound compassionate; not soppy, but kind?

Finding Comfort Elsewhere

One of the most difficult things to navigate during a separation is where to go to for comfort if you have previously sought it out mostly within your relationship with the person you are now separate from, maybe at war with, or even trying to leave. It can feel like there's no school nurse when you've cut your knee. This can be one of the things that makes you feel as if you've made the wrong decision, that you need to go back. This feeling can be awful. You can feel deeply alone as you learn to navigate something painful without a person who has been there for you before.

Some endings allow the continuation of friendship, but make sure you tolerate the loss first before reconnecting, otherwise it can be confusing. We need to move through the pain and really separate in order to come out the other side. Draw other healthy relationships closer at this time; ask for support where you maybe once did not. But be mindful of seeking out potentially destructive closeness that is transient. Know this is temporary – you will reorientate and, just like a cut knee, you need time to sting and scab before you can heal.

WHERE TO FIND COMFORT

Outside of your ex, what people, places and activities bring you comfort?

» Can you get closer to those? For example, telling an old friend your worries, joining a dance class, getting a nice soft blanket, getting a hug from your dad, buying some paints, spending time with a pet?

» Nurture yourself with food (see page 109).

» Don't overload your diary and create space to feel where you are at.

You Are Allowed to Feel It All

This can be a profoundly emotionally disturbing time, regardless of whether or not you did the leaving or ending. Whether or not it was a mutual decision, if there were or are other parties involved and if you have children or dependants, will all impact on how you feel. We have heard of clients being told they shouldn't be upset as they did the leaving, or that they should be happy because they have finally left, and other versions of this toxic, denying and invalidating approach.

When you are inside a separation, divorce or split, you and your partner are the only people who really hold the truth and depth of what is happening. The outside world will make assumptions and voice opinions, but it is only you who has experienced what you have. Nobody else gets to determine, invalidate or decide what you can and can't, or should and should not feel. You should hold on fiercely to your absolute right to feel it all, to change how you feel and to honour whatever it is that comes for you.

What About the Children?

Do not put your children first in the process of deciding to leave. We see many people arriving in therapy having lived with parents who should have ended relationships a long time ago. They endured 'for the kids' and the children – now adults – are able to say how miserable that was, how uninspiring, and how they would much rather a separation had happened. It may not have been easier, but enduring does nothing to educate children on how to live and how to tolerate emotions. Rather, enduring can show them how to repress feelings.

Give children an experience of what it means to be truthful to yourself, to survive the challenges, and how to move through life's struggles. So do not stay for the kids. However, do think about timing things around exams or big life events if you can. Do put your children first in aspects that impact their experiences of something difficult, for example:

» Don't fight in front of children.
» Don't run the other parent down.
» Don't tell lies about each other.
» Don't be a pain with plans.
» Try to champion the other as a parent (help the kids get them birthday/Mother's Day/Father's Day cards, and so on).
» Share information about the kids so they feel held and safe.
» Allow contact that the child needs and wants; don't be divisive.

» Look at old pictures together/talk about the good times you shared and your happy memories.

» Have a family WhatsApp if you can, and if the kids have phones. Share plans and pictures, celebrate the kids' successes, send memes, show that there is still a connection there.

» If you are sad, be sad and don't hide it, but don't seek the child as a caretaker.

» Apologise to your children/ex in front of your children if you have been wrong.

» Keep your promises and plans and be reliable (where you can – it's also important that children can tolerate legitimate let-downs).

» Show kindness and practise softness.

» Do allow children to feel and share feelings without you jumping to defend. Allow them space to have their own experiences and feelings about what is going on and validate and support them.

» Children might need more contact with other people who love them at this time, such as friends, family or godparents. Support that to happen.

» They might need a therapist of their own. Don't take this as a criticism of your parenting – we all need our own space to process (this might be hard for you, but challenge yourself through it).

» Speak to school and let them know what's happening.

» Hold normal boundaries, around behaviour and mealtimes for example, so they feel safe.

How you demonstrate, navigate and lead your children through these big life events is how they will learn to be in the world.

You will not always get it right, and that is perfectly OK. When you notice that, say so: 'I wish I'd done this differently, that can't have been nice', 'This has been on my mind, what could I have done differently?', 'How did that make you feel?', 'I'm sorry, it's been worrying me. I've been thinking about you' are all useful ways to stay connected. Your child will not learn from you pretending to be perfect, or hiding mistakes; they'll learn from how you show them your humanness. This is how they'll get equipped for life – from your reflectiveness and ability to own difficult things. Keeping your growth at the centre shows them what to strive for.

Finding Gratitude

Holding space to honour and find gratitude for the time you and your ex have spent together is a really important part of the separation process. Remember the moments of joy you had, the person you once loved or had affection for, how they impacted your life and what you will miss about being with them. This allows you to grieve for what has been lost and for what is being left behind. If you feel too angry or upset for now to find grati-tude, that's fine, but do try to return to it later.

THINGS THAT CAN HELP WITH SEPARATION AND DIVORCE

1. Write down how you feel, what you want to say and what you wish you had had the opportunity to say.

2. Give yourself time. Take each day and don't rush for solutions or answers – trust in the process, no matter how painful it is.
3. Avoid the blame game. Work on acceptance rather than carrying ill feeling and hatred.
4. Change the way you speak to yourself and be aware of the messages you tell yourself. Big yourself up, back yourself.
5. Talk to others who have been through separation, not for advice specifically, but for sharing, caring and support.

Try Not to Focus On the 'You' But the 'I'

You might become fixated on what the other party has or hasn't done; how they have made you feel or not feel. Instead of focusing on their part in the relationship, it is really helpful to take the focus away from the other and spotlight yourself. Ask yourself:

»   How was I to be with in that relationship? What face did I show? What version of myself did I bring to the table?
»   How would my ex describe me? How does that make me feel?
»   What did I do that was helpful/unhelpful?
»   How could I have done things differently? What have I learnt about myself through this?
»   How did I contribute to the ending?

» What did I really need? Was I able to ask for it? How did I feel when I didn't get it? Was it their job to give it me?

» How will I do things differently with my growth in mind for the future?

Find Space to Talk

Finding ways to stay connected with your ex, even in the midst of the break and beyond, can be very therapeutic. You will particularly need this if you have children or shared assets. However, we would not suggest this for abusive relationships.

We are often told to have a 'clean break', to close the door, and while sometimes this can be helpful – you will know what you need for yourself – there is no one shoe-that-fits-all. Talking things out, understanding yourself through their experience, asking questions and feeling fully heard (or at least fully spoken out) can help a lot for your next relationship.

Don't weaponise the logistics of things that need discussing, such as money, shared property or other assets, invitations to events, animals and particularly children. Using discussions around these as a vehicle to express your emotions/vent anger/take control can become very confusing and challenging for all those involved. Try to come into contact with what you are feeling outside of these interactions. This is very, very hard, but it is really helpful if you can keep negotiations simple and practical when they are about practical things. When they are not, take it to therapy or share it with a friend – with someone else who's been through it – and then think about your approach and how best to handle it. You can then make space to talk about the things you are feeling.

SIDE NOTE

If you are really harbouring hopes of getting get back together and want to explore that, try to face this head-on, rather than dressing it up as an ending meet-up, contact for reasons that really aren't necessary, or drunken phone calls which leave you feeling lonelier. Mixed feelings, or wanting to get back together, can be really difficult to face, but if you feel this way, try to make it more conscious; think about the options you have to support yourself here. Is there mileage in sharing your thoughts with your ex? If so, how? If not, what can you do with these feelings? Perhaps, instead, share with a trusted friend or journal. Or be with the anguish of it rather than deflecting it into miscommunications which can often lead to more confusion and pain.

I (Jodie) worked with a couple in therapy for 20 sessions. They had come to therapy with the hope of ending a 14-year relationship amicably. They had two children. One party was not feeling fulfilled in the relationship and had, in fact, emotionally exited some years before.

The couple arrived in polar positions: one was shut down, afraid to express their deep and heartfelt desires around how much the separation was needed for them. They appeared withdrawn and defensive against the other. The other was angry and upset, not able to articulate what they really wanted to say, because each interaction came across as angry. Our time together was focused on trying to move each of them away from the positions they were holding into some otherness that might liberate them a little, to make things easier for them and the children.

We spent ten sessions reminiscing about their relationship, where they met, how they felt, the ups and the downs, what had attracted them to each other and the silliness that had been a big part of their intimate connection. They told me stories of their younger years, with some laughter and some tears. In the early sessions they spoke to me, but as sessions moved on they spoke to each other: 'Do you remember when . . . ?', 'I love it when you . . .' They were gradually able to look at each other and hold space for what they had been to each other. In doing so they both were able to allow the grief to come. Both had, in their own way, been avoiding it.

The outcome did not change for the relationship – it did end, but they were able to remain in relation to each other in a more useful way. They moved from avoidance to feeling, and in that was deep gratitude and respect for what they had been to each other. Towards the end of the work, we were able to look ahead at how they would co-parent and how they might support one another. There were hugs at the end all round (even for me) and I looked out of the window of the therapy room when they left and watched them cross the road arm-in-arm.

None of what we've covered in this chapter will mitigate your feelings fully – this is an incredibly painful process for some. We are feeling beings, so loss, change and losing connection and connectedness to people we once, and may still, love, can alter us at our core. That can feel unparalleled to anything else we might have experienced before. Don't rush yourself; treat yourself with the love and compassion you so deserve. There are some useful resources on page 320 if you feel you need more support. Be kind in your words to yourself more often than not, and know that love and the loss of relationships is the thing that gets sung and written about most – the pain of it translates across creative mediums for a reason.

Chapter 11

Why We Need to Talk About Grief, Death and Loss

It is in times of grief, perhaps, that we are most strongly confronted with the uncontrollable and unavoidable nature of change. Death is the one change that we all know is coming; it is written into our contract with life from the day we take our first breath. It is, at once, the weirdest and most normal thing that can happen on earth. While there is grief in change, there is also change in grief; change that sweeps across the personal, collective, psychological, physical, social and spiritual plains of our lives.

The first time I (Chance) encountered death was at eight years old. It is a fuzzy memory – I can't quite reach out and grab it, but it lingers, like one of those squiggly lines in the corner of your eye. I was sitting on the stairs of a house that was not mine, and my mum's friend came to me and said: 'Your dad has died.' I'd already overheard from the muffled voices downstairs that he had overdosed. She kept that detail out. Nonetheless, I look back and admire the frankness and succinct delivery of that news, in just four words. Not that 'he has passed away', that we had 'lost him' or 'that he was in a better place' or any of the other euphemisms that aim to soften or confuse death.

What I did not know at the time was that it would never be spoken about again – never uttered. It became a void that grew legs and followed me throughout my childhood, into my adolescence and right up until this day. I think it is because death is something that our culture encourages us to delay, avoid, hide, cheat and deny – though it is present in our lives with as much certainty as the seasons or the passage of time. The death of a parent, a partner, a child, someone we went to school with, a friend, a friend of a friend, death through miscarriage or suicide, death through old age or sudden death . . . All of us at some point will be confronted with it.

If You Are Grieving

In therapy, the first step we would take is noticing and observing: notice if you are grieving. All the phenomena of grieving are familiar – the waves of exhaustion, the sighing, the feelings of emptiness and hopelessness, the shortness of breath, the seductive pull towards the 'other side' to join them in their reality, the 'magical thinking' of turning back the clock and the calendar, to what might have been: 'if only I had . . .' (fill in the blank). Grief looks like sadness, numbness, guilt, shame or self-blame, feeling stuck ('How do I move on?'), your body keeping the score (tension in the jaw, fists and body), questioning of identity ('Who am I now?'), anger, shock, denial or disbelief, bargaining ('Could I have done anything to prevent this?'), anxiety . . . in writing this, we can see the innately human impulse to package very big, messy emotions into neat and tidy points.

These are just a few of the thousand more ways of experiencing grief. No two are the same. No grief process is linear. Each grief map belonging to an individual may echo or mirror the deeply archetypal experience of loss, but when we zoom in on the granular detail, we will notice differences in contours. Each map tracing its own journey. But, in yourself, start by observing. (There are some helpful resources on page 320 if you feel you need to access further support.)

THE 'FIVE STAGES' OF GRIEF

We've had many clients come to us seeking therapy after a bereavement. They will often refer to Elisabeth Kübler-Ross's 'five stages of grief' (denial, anger, bargaining, depression and acceptance) and question where they are along the line. One man even had them printed out, tear-soaked, crumpled in a tightly-gripped hand, voicing: 'But I don't know where I'm at. I should be bargaining now, but I am still so angry. I wish I could just get over it.'

The five stages are ingrained in our collective cultural consciousness as the natural progression of emotions that we can expect to experience after the death of a loved one. Neat, tidy and sequential, they are often interpreted as a compact Ikea-style, flat-pack model of grief that follows a linear journey from denial to acceptance after stopping at anger, bargaining and depression along the way. But they were never meant to be applied to the bereaved or the grieving. Instead, they were founded on conversations Kübler-Ross had with terminally ill patients. She surmised that there were stages of various emotions that the terminally ill would go through after learning about a life-limiting condition. But despite Kübler-Ross being clear about the intention of the five stages, we have held on tightly to them as a script to follow.

As pattern-seeking primates that have used storytelling to evolve, survive and make sense of an often chaotic and unpredictable world, we like order. The stages tell a story; they have a beginning, a middle and an end. They give a narrative to live by: 'you might be feeling this now, but soon . . .'. But this is often the problem: on one side, we might meet validation and encouragement in this, but on the other are expectations, guilt and pressure, mainly experienced by people who do not feel what they think they should.

But grief follows no order and we don't think there ever is a 'getting over it'. Your grief will ebb and it will flow. It will follow its own timeline, its own rhythm that is individual to you, and it certainly never goes entirely away.

Three Alternative Models of Grief

It can be helpful to look at some ways of thinking about grief to anchor you in times when the waves of grief drag you out to sea. Here are three models or theories that honour the reality of the grieving, including the messiness of grief and the endurance it demands. Know that these are theories – use what is helpful and discard the rest.

1. GROWING AROUND GRIEF

(Helpful if you're a griever who cringes at the sentence 'time heals all wounds')
Lois Tonkin's model of growing around grief challenges the idea that 'time heals all wounds' or that 'grief disappears with time'.

Picture a circle: this is you, your life and everything you are experiencing. Now imagine a time when you were in the throes of grief and shade in the circle to represent it. When grieving, we become overwhelmed with it, it fills our experience and we begin to view the world through the lens of aching. We might struggle to sleep, eat and occupy our mind with something else. Grief can feel entirely consuming, which means that the circle becomes completely shaded. Tonkin suggests that instead of the shaded area growing smaller, the outer circle (representing you) begins to grow bigger. Over time, your grief will stay much the same, but your life will begin to grow around it.

This concept is similar to Jung's thoughts in that 'we don't so much solve our problems as we outgrow them. We add capacities and experiences that eventually make us bigger than the problem'. Tonkin's idea is that as we have new lived experiences, make new connections, have new adventures and find moments of meaning again, our lives will begin to grow bigger than our grief. It is a theoretical model that honours grief's longevity and shows us that we will not always be consumed by it; we can still live and grow. It gives permission for grief to be a part of our lives,

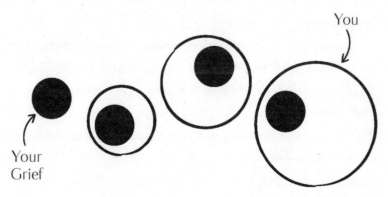

Lois Tonkin's model of grief

2. DUAL PROCESS MODEL

(Helpful if you're a griever who doesn't want to confront your feelings all the time)

Many people talk about grief as something to be tackled head-on and something that must be 'worked through' in order to 'move on from' the loss of a loved one.

As anyone who has ever lost someone they love knows, facing grief head-on can be exhausting. Some days, we just won't be able to. And that's exactly what the dual process model proposes. Stroebe and Schut suggest that when it comes to grief, it is only natural that we distract ourselves and find ways of distancing ourselves from the overwhelming emotions that come with grief. They suggest that there is a time for grief work and a time for grief rest.

What they discovered in their research was that there are two emotional processes/ways of behaving that can be found in human grief – loss-oriented and restoration-oriented – and that people tend to oscillate, jumping back and forth between the two:

Loss-oriented

Things that remind us of the person who has died, or their death, are referred to as 'loss-oriented stressors'. These are thoughts, feelings or actions that lead us to focusing on our grief and pain. This might look like reflecting on how much we miss them, digging out old photos and trinkets or recounting memories of them. Loss-oriented stressors can put us in touch with really strong emotions, deep sorrow, anger and loneliness.

Restoration-oriented

'Restoration-oriented stressors' serve as distractions from our grief and bring us rest from the emotions that come with it. Whether it be throwing ourselves into our work, meals with friends, exercise, walking, doing chores, listening to podcasts or watching something, these activities let us get on with our daily lives and offer temporary distractions and relief from emotional pain.

For prolonged periods, restoration-oriented strategies can be unhealthy. But, Stroebe and Schut stress that alongside loss-orientated stressors, this is a natural and normal way of coping with grief. It's our psyche's way of easing the pain and carrying us through so we can meet daily tasks, look after ourselves and continue to live. Without this submerging back into normality and order, without these moments where we can sign into the ordinary, Stroebe and Schut argue that we could end up not being able to take care of ourselves or get on with our daily lives.

As we grieve, we switch, or 'oscillate', between these two different modes of being. Moving in and out of each one (hence 'dual process'). Stroebe and Schut stress that this is natural and should be embraced, affirming that: 'at times the bereaved will be confronted by their loss, at other times they will avoid memories, be distracted, or seek relief by concentration on other things'. This movement between the two allows for a coming to terms with the reality of the loss in manageable amounts.

This is the part of the dual process model that honours the fact that we never fully 'get over' the death of someone we love. One moment we might be out for dinner with a friend (restoration-oriented) and a song may be playing in the restaurant that reminds us of the person who died (loss-oriented). We might cry at this, savouring the moment and honouring the memory of the deceased and our attachment to them.

What is important in this model is balance. Too much focus on one process can signal maladaptive ways of coping, whether this means being stuck in the all-consuming place of grief, or whether this means avoiding confronting the emotions of a death altogether.

3. CONTINUING BONDS

(Helpful if you're a griever who doesn't want to just 'move on' and 'detach' from the person who has died)

Developed by authors and grief experts Phyllis Silverman, Dennis Klass and Steven Nickman within their book *Continuing Bonds: New Understandings of Grief*, the 'continuing bonds' theory challenges previous, more linear models of grief that end in acceptance, detachment and a new life. Silverman and colleagues argued that it is entirely normal for the bereaved to continue their bond with the person who has died.

In the book, the authors unpack examples of how various cultures mourn, from Japanese people and how they maintain a deep spiritual connection with their ancestors, to the Mexican festival Dìa de los Muertos (Day of the Dead), which celebrates the connection between the living and their ancestors.

Continuing bonds acknowledge that grief is ongoing; even calling it a 'journey' implies that there is an end to it. Grief is something that becomes a part of us. As do those we have lost.

Under this model, when someone we loved dies, the task isn't to work through a series of stages and end at acceptance and building a new life, putting our experience of loss and the memory of the person who has died in a tidy box. Instead, it is about slowly finding a way to recalibrate and redefine our relationship with the person who has died, making space for a continued bond and attachment with that person in a way that will evolve and endure throughout our life, never remaining the same. Rather than assuming detachment as a normal grief response, continuing bonds considers natural human attachment, even in death.

Similar to the loss-orientated process we saw previously, the process of continuing bonds can be found in various ways, such as talking to a loved one at their graveside or resting place, continuing with rituals you used to share together (a regular walk, eating a favourite meal, singing a favourite song), keeping small keepsakes to remember them by, honouring them through fundraising or charity work, or just quite simply remembering special moments with them.

Despite so many of these behaviours being familiar to those who are bereaved, many are still met with expectations, perhaps delivered through bewildering comments like: 'Are you still sad about that? But it was ages ago', 'You're still young; you will find someone else', 'They were old; at least they lived a long life.' These statements are the source of so much shame. But we should take comfort in knowing that being connected seems to facilitate the bereaved person's ability to cope with loss and the accompanying changes in their lives.

Our task with all grief is to make space for processing and observing; that is all we can do. There is no timeline for this and there is no one, or best, way to do it, but know that you do not have to do it alone. Reach out to those you can. The reality is that we will grieve forever. It ebbs and flows. It comes and goes. We do not 'get over' the loss of a loved one; we learn to live with it. Sit with it. Cry with it. Dance with it. Distract yourself from it. Remind yourself of it. You will heal and you will rebuild yourself around the loss you have suffered. You will be whole again but you will never be the same. Nor should you be the same nor would you want to be. What you once enjoyed and deeply loved you can never fully lose, for all that you love deeply becomes part of you.

WHAT TO SAY (AND NOT SAY) TO A GRIEVING PERSON

Knowing the right thing to say to someone grieving doesn't come naturally to most of us. Our culture generally avoids speaking about death, dying or grieving. For this reason, we aren't able to sharpen our skills in talking to those who have lost someone they love.

Unhelpful things you should not say

Let's start with some unhelpful examples we have come across from our clients, and people who have contacted us through social media:

» 'Be strong.'

» 'Stop crying.'

» 'I understand how you feel.'

» 'At least they are in a better place; their suffering is over.' (Actually, just don't start any sentence with 'at least'. It is probably not going to be helpful. There is no silver lining, just acknowledge how bloody awful and painful the situation is and validate their feelings.)

» 'Aren't you over them yet? They have been dead for a while now.'

» 'You're young; you can still have other children.'

» 'You're young; you will find someone else.'

» 'God's in charge. God doesn't give us more than we can handle.'

Helpful things you could say

» 'What can I take off your plate?'

» 'How do you wish people would act around you right now?'

» 'What do you wish people to know about what you are going through?'

» If you have one, share a memory of the person who they lost.

» Offer them space to talk.

» Recognise how hard it is for them.

» Be active in suggesting how you can help.

Sometimes you don't need to say anything. When it comes to helping someone who is grieving, here's the thing: you do not need to make it better. The most basic and powerful way to support another person in grief is to listen. Just listen.

Some Final Thoughts on Death

Talking about death does not bring it closer. A cloak-wearing, scythe-carrying Grim Reaper does not just suddenly appear to take us off. Instead, talking about death turns our grief into something shareable and communal. It doesn't have to be morbid; it can be cathartic and releasing. Existential psychotherapist Irvin D. Yalom thinks about death as something to be faced like any other fear: through familiarisation, dissecting it and analysing it enough to the point that we can properly comprehend it. Only then can we free this fear and focus on living a life devoid of regret.

Talking about death prepares us, reduces shock and allows us to truly and fully live. Don't shy away from it.

Chapter 12

Parenting and Your Mental Health

Becoming a parent can be an incredible, joyous, hideous and terrifying time. It's a time of change, when old wounds can resurface, we can feel not good enough and we can feel tremendous pressure to live up to our own positive childhoods or not become our own parents. You might experience pressure to prove your abilities and feel judged by those around you. You might find that depression sets in, anxiety is high or relationships that were good are suddenly floundering. You might feel let down by friends or feel a disconnect from loved ones or a partner. You might be grieving the old version of you, feel overwhelmed by the task at hand and sleep-deprived, all at the same time as being told repeatedly how lucky you are and what a wonderful time it is! Of course, you might also feel overwhelming love, contentedness, purpose and invigoration for life. You might feel a mixture of it all at different times, all the while with another human (or humans) to tend to.

Though society can, and does appear to, champion the 'perfect' parent, it is so important to give space to the parts of you that are struggling with parenting or even wishes they could not be a parent just for a minute or maybe even turn the clock back. It's so important for our growth that we find ways to allow it all. Think about those stages of change we've already talked about: honour the loss, make space for the grieving, give room to that awkward in-between where one hand is on the past and one hand is on the future; one hand on parenthood, one hand on your past self. Notice what parts of your experience are calling you to face them – the sadness, the hope, the anticipation, the gradual acceptance. Adjustment can, and will, come. (See page 320 for a list of some helpful resources if you feel you need more support.)

The minute I (Jodie) think about the topic of parenting, I immediately think about Sadie, who was six when I began working with her. Her mum (who was a teenager when she had Sadie), had made numerous attempts to try to parent successfully, but Sadie always ended up back in care. I was only working with the child in this case and was given the brief to support her as she had presented 'disturbing' behaviour at school.

I was part of a meeting focused on a set of tasks and objectives the mother had to adhere to in order to keep Sadie with her at home. The ramifications if she didn't were that her daughter would be placed in longer-term care. I was sitting directly opposite the mother and observed that she looked very stressed – she was twiddling her hands, looking at the floor, shallow breathing, and had a cap pulled down low and a massive coat on. We adjourned for a break and I found myself alone with her in the room. She sat quietly, looking at her feet. I asked her how she was doing. She said, 'I feel terrible.' I asked her what it was she really needed right now, and she looked at me and said, 'Nobody has ever asked me if I want my daughter.' So I asked her, 'Do you want your daughter?' and she said, 'At the moment, no.' I told her that must be hard and, at that point, I could almost see the weight lift from her.

It transpired, in fact, that this was the last time Sadie went into care. I was able to encourage the family therapist to work with the mother on the part of her that really didn't want to be a parent. This enabled her to change, to feel validated and not judged, which in turn enabled her to parent in the best way she could. I saw both the mum and daughter some years later at the bus stop holding hands.

I share this story because I think the most powerful thing we can do as parents is connect to the resistant parts about parenting – the failing, broken bits, the parts we find boring, awful and hard – and allow them space and time. Parenting might be, and often is, a continual struggle for our own autonomy and the desire to care for another. These things are often in opposition and can create great internal friction. Couple this with any unresolved issues from our own childhoods, and it's no wonder that as parents we're often hanging by a thread.

Parenting is a conscious but also an unconscious time. You are consciously in a close relationship with another human who needs looking after, feeding, loving and showing the ropes to, and one who you will come face-to-face with yourself through.

You'll come up against your own anger, frustration, sadness, limitations, and yourself as a child – the best and the broken parts. You'll also unconsciously come into contact with parts of yourself you've never met as you've not been a parent before.

Your mental health might flounder at different points in your child's development, and that is to be expected. Some feelings will be connected to the huge amounts of growth you are both going through and some will be connected to your own experiences as an infant, many of which you won't be conscious of. You'll sometimes find the experience of being a parent impossible, sometimes incredible, and sometimes you'll feel deep shame at the way you behave.

> Parenting is a time when so much care,
> compassion and nurturing is needed,
> not just for the child but for you, too.

Be gentle with yourself. Know that it's OK to want to run away. It's OK to be bored, disillusioned and overwhelmed. It's OK not to always feel gushing love for being a parent.

HOW TO TAKE CARE OF YOUR MENTAL HEALTH WHEN PARENTING FEELS TOO MUCH

1. Don't be afraid to tell people how hard it's feeling, if it is.
2. Avoid comparing yourself to others – comparison is rife in the parenting world.

3. Carve out space and time just for yourself.

4. Don't overload yourself with reading material on how to parent as this can make you feel as if you are falling short.

5. Reflect on what's happening for you and how you're feeling about being a parent.

6. Notice behaviour patterns in the way you parent that don't make you feel good and tend to them.

7. Try not to take it out on the kids – notice when and if you do, and apologise.

8. Try to engage with your own childhood at the same age as your infant. If you can, talk to your parents about yourself as a child, look at pictures, and notice what feels similar and what feels different about the experience.

9. Practise holding on and letting go (see page 177).

10. Ask yourself often: 'What am I doing well and what needs attention here?'

Becoming and being a parent is one of the most complex life phases. As we saw in Chapter 4, we are all the products of our own parents' journeys and this is something that prevails. Evolution means we adapt and progress. Maybe we will not make the same mistakes as our parents, but we will make some – it's how our children will evolve to be better than us.

Every single person arrives in the therapy room with something to say about their own childhood and you will be no different. Keep an open mind and an open heart and champion a desire to give it your best – to break generational patterns of dysfunction and keep a mirror up to yourself in a way that perhaps your parents did not.

TIME FOR REFLECTION

Becoming a parent can be difficult and it is often a time when mental health issues come to the surface. Try to keep yourself as conscious as possible around what might be happening for you at this time. Some things to think about are:

» What are your experiences of parenting from your childhood?

» What worked and what didn't?

» How do you feel about other parents in your circle? Are you fiercely judging, do you have compassion or are you feeling something else?

» What are your fears about parenting? What are your hopes?

» If you are a parent, how do you think your children would or will describe you? How does that make you feel?

» What support do you have available to you and do you need more?

I (Jodie) remember when my own son was born, telling my clinical supervisor that I was worried I was going to fuck up being a parent. And she said, 'The fact you are even asking me that is a very good sign that you will not.' I suspect my kids would argue otherwise, but there is something powerful in us being here together and even wondering, considering what we might do to make it better. Keep positive growth happening. That you have consideration enough to read this chapter is a good sign that you want to be different.

PART 4

Being Human

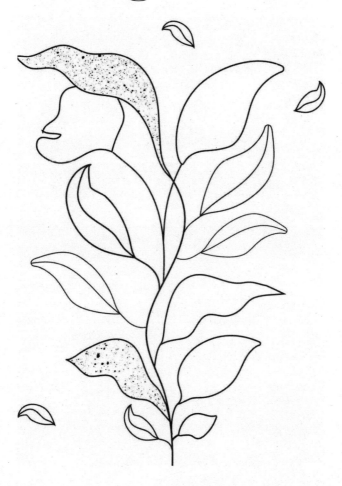

In reality, we can do little to fully prepare ourselves for some of the challenges we will endure during our time on this earth. We can do little to prepare ourselves for all of the suffering we will encounter, inside ourselves and in others. We can do little to prepare for when things don't go according to plan; for when we can't find the words, for when our unmet needs drive our behaviour in ways we aren't aware of, for when life feels unfair and unjust, for when people let us down, and for when things inevitably change or come to an end.

Because of this, when it comes to navigating relationships, trusting others, believing we are enough, communicating effectively, understanding ourselves, honouring our potential and feeling relatively authentic, confident and unashamed, we struggle.

In this section, we'll touch upon each of these struggles. Not in an attempt to solve or to fix them; not to help you 'hack' them, 'unlock' or find ways to 'fast-track' your way out of any difficult emotions that come with them, but to make space for them. All we need for this is to be curious. To open ourselves up to the possibility that we don't fully know ourselves, that there are hidden bits that are even hidden from ourselves.

To us, this is what 'being human' and what growth is all about. It is being open to the full length, breadth and depth of our experiences, especially the hard ones. It is not about every-thing being perfect or about being happy all of the time; it is about paying particular attention to the things we find tough, the repeated patterns of behaviour that keep us stuck, the same old roads we keep walking down, the same holes we keep fall-ing into and the thinking traps we get ensnared in. It is about paying attention and then bringing to consciousness. Which is the most essential, but under-celebrated and underrated part of any self-development journey.

Chapter 13

Navigating Relationships

Relationships are a key component of the work that happens in the rooms at Self Space. Our relationship with ourselves, and then all the others in our life, form the foundation for our mental wellness. Almost all clients come to us with challenges in how they are relating to themselves and subsequently others. This often takes the initial shape of 'they are treating me like . . .' or 'I don't get on with them because they are . . .' Our work in the room is to orientate everything back to you. What is it that you are responsible for, both in the relationship to yourselves and the others in your life? What themes can you notice, what roles do you play and what challenges do you face regularly? What can this teach us about you and how you relate to others?

When our house is in order, our relationships feel, in the most part, good (this does not mean perfect). This contributes to a sense of well-being, less drama, less high emotion, more feelings of positivity and being supported, being seen and heard . . . and all of these things make unavoidable mental health challenges easier to navigate.

Romantic Relationships

Growing up, we learn how to relate to others. We look to the adults in our lives to learn what family, relationships and love look like. As we saw in Chapter 4, we unconsciously mine the data from our parents/caregivers and internalise how they relate to us: how much they make space for our emotions, how independent they let us be, how consistent they are. Sometimes this sets us up for healthy relationships; other times, we end up with a blueprint that invariably causes us a lot of pain. Then, as adults, we use the information from these relationships as a guide to choose a partner. It seems absolutely nonsensical that as adults, we seek out the kind of familial and childhood 'love' that caused pain, but as repetition compulsion predicts, we will find anyone who displays a similar type of love and regard to our parents/caregivers incredibly magnetising and intoxicatingly appealing. Repetition compulsion is commonly, and often unconsciously, hoping that the outcome may be different.

JOURNAL PROMPTS

Free-write and reflect on these questions:

» What are the three things that you needed the most when you were younger?

» Were they provided?

» What are you looking for in a romantic partner emotionally? (Try to be truthful with yourself when answering this question.)

» Do any of these needs overlap with your childhood needs?

» What have your romantic partners had in common?

The blueprint for how we bond and attach to others starts from birth and continues through childhood. It can be traced to our dependence on someone else for our safety, security, belonging and, fundamentally, our survival. This is usually our primary caregiver/parent. This need for survival is the foundation of human attachment, so when our safety is under threat, for example, when we experience trauma, we naturally look to someone seen as a caregiver in our lives, someone who provides consistency, support, protection and care.

If you experienced abuse or neglect from a caregiver who also loved you, then you can learn to associate love with abuse. This becomes the template for how you learn to relate to others and form relationships.

Something life-defining and deeply intimate,
often not for the better, is over when the child
speaks what their parent could not. This
is how cycles of trauma begin to change.

TIME FOR REFLECTION

» What ideas of the world do you have that you learnt from your parents?

» How can you honour some of these experiences?

» How can you let go of some of the less useful ones in your day to day? (Ask yourself whether you're playing these out in your everyday life.)

RELATIONSHIP RUTS

In the therapy room, we commonly hear statements like:

» 'What's wrong with me? I'm an intelligent, attractive person with a successful career. I have loads to offer, but I keep picking partners who treat me like shit.'

» 'A few weeks into dating this person, and I'm already making myself miserable worrying that she doesn't find me attractive enough. So I'll probably do the same with this one as last time and turn my fear of not being good enough into a self-fulfilling prophecy and ruin yet another chance at a decent relationship.'

» 'Why do I keep repeating patterns?'

The truth is that humans are creatures of habit, and habits come from repetition: what we did yesterday, we will do today. This is just as true for falling into the same relationship ruts. We find comfort in repetition and routines, even when they have the potential of disrupting or distressing us.

We're comfortable with familiar old patterns, even when they cause us stress or pain. So, it's no surprise that we continue to repeat them, even when they don't get us where we want to go. How many of us have stayed in relationships that we know are unhealthy, with a person who's repeatedly hurt us?

> Life is too short to stay in a relationship
> that no longer serves either of you.

The neuroscience of behaviour tells us that neurons in our brain like familiar pathways and routines, just as much as our emotions do. Neural pathways (that transmit information to the rest of our body) are created based on our habits and repetitive behaviour.

Picture this: Imagine that you're going on a walk and decide to go off the designated route. You venture through overgrown grass, move aside branches and walk through bushes to find your way to your destination. Once you decide you've gone far enough, you turn back and follow the same path you just made to return to the route you were on – the one where the overgrown grass has become flatter and worn down. It wouldn't make a huge amount of sense to struggle through, creating another route. Over time, as other people travel down the way you have created, it becomes a well-worn pathway. Walking routes are similar to your neural pathways – once a path is carved through the 'overgrown' grass, the neurons begin to follow it.

With a little bit of understanding around what makes us tick, we can develop and strengthen new neural pathways and begin to build a road map to change the way we approach and navigate our relationships.

SIDE NOTE

There will be some of you reading this who will, devastatingly, find yourself in, or have been in, an abusive relationship in which you are *absolutely not* complicit in the circumstances you find yourself. Please take what you need and what feels relevant, and leave the rest. (See page 320 for a list of some helpful resources where you can access support.)

Accept the part you play in the dynamic

It is much easier for us to ring our friends, let them rally around, support us and bask in echoes of: 'they were a dickhead anyway' than it is to be aware of, and understand, the role we might play in our painful and unhealthy relationships. We have to have the guts to change what we have been doing in the past to make space for new experiences for us. This is not about berating ourselves or hitting ourselves on the back with the whip of self-blame and shame, but about accepting our part in the relationship, however small, to retain some agency and autonomy.

FIVE WAYS TO STOP REPEATING PATTERNS IN RELATIONSHIPS

Growing up, we learn what love looks like. As adults, we use these relationship models as a guide to pick a partner. (See Chapter 4 for more on understanding what has gone before and how this impacts the present.) Take a look at the points below to help you identify your relationship patterns, and how you might make changes:

1. Reflect on your childhood: What did you need most in your childhood? How did your parents respond to these needs? Are you looking for your romantic partners to meet the same needs?
2. Accept your part: You have to be willing to change what you have been doing in the past in order to create an experience that feels completely new to you. Blaming yourself is not helpful but accepting your part in a relationship dynamic is essential.
3. Examine expectations: Normal relationships are a far cry from those in TV, films and books. A healthy relationship isn't built on constant excitement and emotional curveballs (which is actually exhausting). What are your favourite love stories? What are the 'truths' you took away? How do they inform your expectations?
4. Be aware of trauma bonds: In trauma bonding, we repeat abusive, neglectful or traumatic childhood experiences from our caregivers and this becomes the blueprint for how we attach to others. Notice if

you try to make the best of a bad relationship or if you continue to seek contact with that person despite knowing they will cause further pain.

5. Focus on what you can control: Remember, you are in control of yourself, your own choices, actions and behaviours. We can shift the dynamic and outcome of the relationship by changing our half of the interaction.

TIME FOR REFLECTION

There is a wonderful question from Jerry Colona that we encourage you to ask yourself: 'How have I been complicit in creating the conditions I say I don't want?'

Now, complicit is the important word here. It says 'not completely responsible but I am accepting my part'. By doing this, we begin to take responsibility for our mistakes – until we do that, nothing can change.

Assess your expectations about romantic relationships

Disney, sitcoms, teenage novels and corny Hollywood films have all gone a long way in causing us to have unrealistic expectations regarding relationships on a mass scale. Look at the Disney princesses:

» Cinderella: dancing with the Prince at a party for a couple of hours and being convinced he was the love of her life.
» Ariel: changing her whole self just to fit into 'his' world.

» Princess Jasmine: being lied to the entire time, and still choosing to marry him.

» Belle: grateful for the books but ignoring that he was still her captor.

In films, we're always shown the moment of falling in love, but never the work that goes into maintaining that love. Instead, we are captivated by the slow motion, the shallow depth of field, the close-up and music, the rollercoaster of emotions, the last-minute plot changes and grand gestures – these things don't often happen in real life. Nonetheless, so many of us fall into the trap of comparing our relationships to these stories, which causes us to mistake security and consistency in our partner as being boring and over-predictable.

Healthy relationships are not built on running-through-the-airport excitement and emotional curveballs; these things are exhausting. Instead, when we find ourselves in a properly secure relationship, we can take comfort in the fact that our partner is going to be there with us through all of the shit.

JOURNAL PROMPT

Think about all of the films, books and sitcoms you watched growing up:

» What did they teach you about love?

» What plots were common?

» What are your favourite love stories?

» Do any of them connect to your expectations of romantic relationships?

Identify trauma bonds

If you feel stuck and powerless in a relationship (including friendships and work relationships), but try to make the best of it, you may be caught up in a trauma bond. If you continue to seek contact with that person despite knowing they will cause you further pain, if you know they are 'sometimes' abusive, but you focus on the 'good' in them, if you find yourself defending the relationship if others criticise it, this may be a trauma bond. Being unable to retreat from an unhealthy relationship can be paralysing and deeply painful.

Here are some of the signs you might be in a trauma bond:

» Obsessing about people who have hurt you, though they are long gone.

» Continuing to seek contact with people whom you know will cause you further pain.

» Going 'overboard' to help people who have been destructive to you.

» Continuing to be a 'team member' when obviously things are becoming destructive.

» Continuing attempts to get people to like you, though they are clearly using you.

» Trusting people again and again who have proven to be unreliable.

» Being unable to retreat from unhealthy relationships.

» Wanting to be understood by those who clearly do not care.

» Choosing to stay in conflict with others, though it would cost you nothing to walk away.

» Persisting in trying to convince people there is a problem and they won't listen.

» Remaining loyal to people who have betrayed you.

» Being attracted to untrustworthy people.

» Being forced to keep damaging secrets about exploitation or abuse.

» Maintaining contact with an abuser who acknowledges no responsibility.

Trauma bonds refer to the attachment bond that is created through repeated abusive, neglectful or traumatic childhood experiences. This relationship pattern becomes internalised as a learnt pattern of behaviour for attachment. When you are trauma bonding, it is easy to mistake abuse as love and not let go. They occur in very toxic relationships and tend to be strengthened by fleeting moments of connection – or at least the hope of something better to come – that we desperately try to hold on to.

We can see how trauma bonds occur: when the person we call our 'significant other', the 'caregiver', is also the one creating trauma by threatening our safety through abusive or neglectful behaviour. Given that it is so naturally ingrained within us from birth to turn to an attachment figure when our safety is under threat, it makes sense that we would turn to our romantic partners when abuse occurs, even if they are the ones who are being abusive to us. This leads to us feeling bonded to them. This is particularly prominent if we have lost friends or strong relationships with others due to being in such a relationship.

SEVEN WAYS TO RETREAT FROM A TRAUMA BOND

1. Commit to living in reality. When you find yourself fantasising about what could be, or what you hope it could be, stop. Even if you don't choose to get out of the relationship straight away, take time to notice how the relationship makes you feel in the present, now. Pay attention to your emotions and see how it is affecting you.

2. Live one decision at a time and one day at a time. Don't scare yourself with 'all-or-nothing' thinking. Don't be too hard on yourself if it takes time to find the strength to leave the relationship.

3. Make decisions that support your self-care (see page 124). Ground your choices in what you feel will be good for you. When you aren't able to do this, talk to yourself in compassionate, understanding and reflective ways.

4. Feel and be with your emotions. Whenever you are away from the toxic relationship and feel an urge to reach out to them, pause. Write down your feelings instead. For example, 'I'm feeling ____. I miss and wish I could be with ____. Instead, right now, I am going to sit and journal my feelings. I am going to lean into the discomfort and untangle myself from the hook, rather than turning to ____.'

5. Allow space for grief. Letting go of a toxic relationship and doing the work around a trauma bond is

so incredibly hard you cannot do it without honouring the reality that you are losing something precious
to you.

6. Understand the 'hook'. Identify what, exactly, you
   are losing. It may be a fantasy, a dream, a promise
   from your partner at the beginning of the relationship to meet and fulfil an unmet need. What about
   the person was so strongly attractive to you?

7. Build healthy connections. A good way to really
   free yourself from unhealthy connections is to start
   investing in healthy ones (see page 172). Develop
   other close, connected and healthy bonded relationships that are not centred on drama. Make these your
   'go-to' people. Take stock of the people around you
   who show you love and support – hang around with
   them as often as you can; bring them close.

Focus on the things that you can control

The only thing that we have control over is ourselves; our
decisions, our actions and our behaviours. We can't completely
control the outcome of our relationships.

'When we are no longer able to change a situation –
we are challenged to change ourselves'
Viktor E. Frankl

While we can't always choose our feelings, we can always choose
how we respond. As Victor Frankl puts it: forces beyond our

control can take away everything we possess except one thing –
our freedom to choose how we will respond to the situation. One
way of taking control over the dynamics of our relationships is
by taking control of our responses and focusing on the type of
person we want to be. We can shift the dynamic and outcome of
relationships by changing our half of the interaction, modelling
what we want and not settling for less.

JOURNAL PROMPT

» What are your three biggest needs in relationships?
» Is there a way of first meeting these needs yourself?
» Can anyone outside of romantic relationships meet
  them?

When you feel out of control or overwhelmed within a relationship, when you feel flooded with emotion, use the STOP
acronym:

» **S**top.
» **T**ake a step back.
» **O**bserve and take stock.
» **P**roceed mindfully.

As psychotherapist and relationship expert, Esther Perel, says,
'The quality of our lives is determined by the quality of our
relationships.' This is because relationships really are one of

the most human experiences. When we play an active role in breaking relationship patterns that don't benefit us, we give ourselves a better shot at growth and finding (and keeping) a healthy long-term relationship.

EMOTIONAL CARETAKING

There's a big difference between caring for others and being an 'emotional caretaker'. Emotional caretaking can be traced right back to our early childhoods. As a small child, your environment is almost entirely made up of the person taking care of you and conditions closely connected to them. If your caregivers had limited support from others, limited access to professional services (such as health visitors or GPs), limited social connections, worries about housing, food or finances, experiences of mental ill health and a high number of adverse childhood experiences (see page 73), your experience might have been one in which your needs were not consistently met.

If this becomes a regular state for a sustained amount of time, to continue to feel safe, you as the child will do anything you have to do to make your caregiver feel better, so that you feel better. This is when compulsive caregiving starts. There is an unconscious role reversal that happens – caretaking acts as a substitute for the missing caregiving, and this dynamic becomes the child's environment and the primary condition for safety. This gets internalised as a rule for relating to people and, as an adult, this translates into a deep need to rescue, fix and take care of others in order to establish a sense of safety and connection.

JOURNAL PROMPT

Have you played the role of emotional caretaker for others?

» What role did you play in your family?

» Have you ever felt the responsibility or impulse to caretake, but then resented others for it?

» What unspoken contracts might be operating in your life: between you and life or between you and family members?

» What are you willing to do differently to own your power and give others their power back, even if it is uncomfortable or painful?

Emotional caretaking involves feeling the chronic responsibility or impulse to caretake others, before yourself. It looks like rushing in to 'solve' the problems or 'fix' the suffering of others. The caretaker role often develops as a result of unspoken family contracts and ends up being a blueprint for how we operate in our adult relationships.

Perhaps you've been made to prevent or fix or rescue people from their feelings in order to help them regulate or remain attached to them. Perhaps your sense of self and worth is found in being of service to others as a result of your needs going unmet by caregivers. Perhaps without supporting others you feel overwhelmed by your own problems. Emotional caretaking looks like:

» Rushing to fix others' feelings.

» Helping others before helping yourself.

» Avoiding conflict to save people from hurt.
» Avoiding saying no because people will be angry.
» Trying to control situations to secure your own comfort.
» People-pleasing to avoid discomfort.
» Jumping into problem-solving as a way of fixing the big feelings.
» Saving or rescuing people from their feelings.
» Denying your own feelings by focusing on helping others.

The primary challenge in all relationships, whether between parents and children, or between life partners, is to honour the 'otherness' of the other. What this means is to have the courage to take on the largeness of our own journey without asking our partners, children or friends to bear it for us. It is the gift of honouring the 'other' in their separateness, their 'otherness'.

It seems paradoxical but true intimacy is really only possible when we fully own our own separateness and honour that in the other – their right to be 'other', to be utterly and totally themselves.

How to release from the role of the caretaker
Releasing the 'emotional caretaker' role takes gritty effort. We'd welcome you to start the work on this by writing two 'no-send' letters:

» One, addressed to your caregiver, starting with: 'Some of the things that I didn't get from you when I was younger, but things that I needed were . . .'
» And one to yourself as a child, validating those things that were missing, starting with: 'As an adult, when I'm looking

back at you now, what I can see is . . ., what I notice is . . ., what I feel is . . .'.

Releasing from the caretaker role is about being in compassionate dialogue with the parts of yourself that might feel unsafe. It takes conscious practice, and includes:

» Not rushing in to 'solve' the problems or 'fix' the suffering of others. Instead, just being present with them.
» Letting people have their upsets instead of rushing in to comfort, explain or apologise (especially if their upset is about their own stuff).
» Allowing people to have their misconceptions of you without feeling a compulsive need to correct them and make them understand you/where you're coming from.
» Walking away from people and situations when it's clear they are not for your highest good (even when they are pleading for help).
» Risking external disapproval for making the choices you know in your heart are right for you.
» Setting boundaries with people or situations that want more of your time and energy than you are willing to give.
» Taking care of and validating yourself, your body, your ideas and your feelings when other people are unable to support you because of their own wounds.

Relationships at Work

Just as we take our professional experience with us into every job, we also take our relational experience. This is made up of our early childhood relationships with our parents or care-givers, our families, our community, the place we grew up in and our romantic and non-romantic relationships. In it are belief systems that we created to survive the challenges of our childhood: beliefs around conflict/repair, fairness/unfairness, self-reliance/trusting others, success/failure, attitudes towards work, money, endings, authority figures and so much more. None of this gets left at the door – we carry it all with us into work.

It's not something any of us learn in school or come into our working lives prepared to even see, much less navigate, but work becomes the stage upon which we play out and replay what has happened to us in our lives – our inner dramas and our relational scripts. Our boss, business partners, managers, colleagues, clients . . . we unconsciously cast them as characters from our past. By doing this, we can find that we actually become complicit in recreating the conditions that allow us to repeat these dynamics.

I (Chance) worked with Sarah (32), a creative director working within an advertising agency. Sarah had come to therapy after feeling overwhelmed and anxious about work. She was exhausted and expressed a creative block, feelings of uncertainty around her job security and feeling not good enough. Sarah found it excruciating being in the unknown and not receiving regular feedback from her managers. She described living in constant fear of being fired. This undermined her confidence and self-esteem and stopped her from feeling creative.

We spent the early parts of the work exploring her anxiety and beginning to try to challenge some of the assumptions she was holding about her not-good-enoughness. We looked at what she was ruminating over about the termination of her employment. We moved in and out of existential reflections before arriving at traumatic moments in Sarah's childhood.

After a difficult transition into a new school at the age of 14, Sarah began to get into trouble. One evening, Sarah's parents locked her out of the house when she did not make curfew. They stopped giving her money and they called the police when she stole from them. She was arrested and put in a 'secure custody facility'. She then lived in supported housing until the age of 15. Tired, exhausted and in need of support, eventually Sarah called her parents and asked to go back home. Her parents let her know that she was able to go back on the condition that she worked hard, got her head down and finished school with good behaviour. Sarah excelled at school and the whole family did not speak of any of this again.

Sarah carried this experience into her adult life where it displaced and projected on to work and her relationships there. She carried her worry and anxiety around being kicked out of the place that offered safety and belonging, and a powerful drive to overwork, as a means of feeling secure and enough. Work became the stage for home (safety, security and belonging). Her boss was cast as the parent: she held a preoccupation with what his thoughts were about her, if he liked her and whether he thought she was doing a good-enough job. One week, Sarah had been called in for a meeting with her boss and she was convinced that she was going to be fired. Instead, her boss voiced that he thought she was doing a fantastic job and that she was getting a promotion. At this moment, the projection shattered. It was only with this very contrasting story – one of validation and affirming feedback – that Sarah was able to let go of the one she was conjuring from her past and playing out in the present.

Sarah was able to make these connections in a way that enabled her to untangle herself from the story being played out, and also gain insight into what she was still carrying from her childhood. She turned these reflections into action and was able to calibrate herself towards making positive changes in her relationship with her parents. Sarah was later able to bridge the work she did in therapy towards her relationship with her mum. The working through of the conflict at work made a lot of space for this to happen.

We've all had relationships at work that we carry with us to our pillows at night, lying there with clenched fists and gritted teeth, seething over this person who makes us miserable and who is probably sleeping like a baby. We might play out arguments and scenarios in which our voices are heard, our points are made and we really stick it to them. But we often don't take a minute to stop and think about the part we might play in this. Whether we like it or not, we carry all of our relational habits with us when we walk through the office door (or open our laptops).

There are lots of hidden dimensions under relationship impasses at work: from power to control, to recognition and respect, to fear and confidence. When conflict happens, it serves us to ask ourselves which dimension is at play. It serves us to first address the immediate. It may feel safer to gossip about a meeting or walk out pissed off than to say: 'When I'm not listened to in a meeting, it makes me feel undervalued and unimportant.' But, keeping it in the 'I', not attacking with 'you', saying it how it is, can go a long way to improving our relationships at work.

And then you can go deeper in your thinking. Ask yourself: what situations from my past am I playing out? Bettering your work life starts with bettering your communication. The better your relationships at work, the better your work.

JOURNAL PROMPTS

- » What am I not saying that needs to be said?
- » What needs asking that I have not asked yet?
- » Who are you, independent of any work identity?

Positive Relationships

We can be so hyper-alert to relationship red flags, noticing and concerning ourselves with the charged relationships in our lives, the ones that cause us concern, that we can neglect the ones that are positive. 'Red flag' relationships can take up a lot of our emotional capacity, meaning we expend less energy, focus and time on those relationships that *are* working – the ones that replenish us, keep us grounded, feel calm and untroublesome; the ones that feel comfortable while also challenging and encouraging our growth and the growth of the relationship.

Relationships that feel good are so important for our life journey. That does not mean there will not be conflict or bumps in the road, but these are negotiable; we can practise our boundaries within them and say how we really feel without fear of abandonment or rejection. We can express our upset or disappointment and feel listened to. This does not mean the relationship is without work, but you have confidence in them. They raise you up when you need it, call you out when you think you don't, champion your successes and help your life to feel better. Make space to notice these relationships.

JOURNAL PROMPT

» Which people or relationships come to mind when you think of positive relationships?

» What works within them?

» How do they differ from those that don't?

GREEN FLAGS IN RELATIONSHIPS

We spend so much time looking out for the red flags in relationships that we forget to look out for green flags. Here are a few signs that you might be on to a good thing. What would you add?

» Instead of playing games, they follow through, call when they say they are going to call and show up to things they said they'd go to.
» You feel able to be open, acknowledge feelings and practise being vulnerable.
» These people have a stable life outside of you. They have other friends or hobbies and don't need or want to spend every minute with you.
» They give you the benefit of the doubt if they think something is up and ask you about it.
» They can practise repair after an argument.
» They demonstrate a commitment to helping you be a better person, while working on themselves equally.
» They never make you feel embarrassed or ashamed when you're with them.
» They take the time to understand what you're feeling when you are upset.
» They know that it is not needy to say what you need.

Loneliness Can Feel Really Shit: Here's What to Do About It

Just as unhealthy relationships and attachments can cause us pain and limit our growth, so too can a lack of authentic connection. Over 9 million people in the UK – almost a fifth of the population – say they are always, or often, lonely. Loneliness tricks us into thinking we are the only one that feels it, but every human on the planet has experienced moments of loneliness and aloneness.

Sometimes, these feelings of loneliness move through us as quickly as the wind, but other times, they linger like a thick fog that we can't see our way out of. Feeling lonely is horrible. It can feel like a hopeless numbness that appears when we need it least. Loneliness can be sneaky; it dresses up as demotivation, boredom, frustration or sadness. Loneliness can remind us how unlovable we are, encourage us to jump on the treadmill of distracting behaviour, pushing others further away, seeking transient contact from multiple sexual partners or interaction with friends who don't really care. It might show up as going to events or places that aren't very safe, using drugs and booze when we are seeking immediate relief and some kind of connection . . . All of which promote a false sense of connection. Not the real stuff but an actual active avoidance with the thing you are seeking deeply, which is intimacy.

No matter where you are on this planet, please know
that you have got company. You are not alone.

Feelings of loneliness often have nothing to do with the number of people around us. You might be standing in busy rooms, whizzing around a party, surrounded by people, but still feel totally alone. We read an article written by a famous frontman in a band who said he spent nine years feeling as if he was on a deserted island, totally alone. When he looks back at pictures of his years on tour, at festivals and events, he can only remember how alone he was. He remembers nothing of others, not even his bandmates.

Lonely feelings mostly come from a lack of authentic connection. When you feel unseen, unheard and disconnected, you feel alone. It is inevitable that all of us have experienced or will experience feeling lonely at one time or another, whether it's a brief pang of being left out of an invite or the more long-term sense of lacking a close relationship – we have all been there. Life-changing events, such as moving to a new place, starting or losing a job, transitioning between college and university, suffering bereavement, chronic illness, separation/divorce, becoming a parent or having fertility struggles, can all make you feel alone. Have you felt alone during times like these?

Loneliness impacts us physically in our stress responses, and with a weakened immune system, higher levels of cortisol and lower levels of oxytocin. It also wounds us psychologically. It ensnares us in a trap many of us struggle to get out of, in that it distorts our perceptions, making us believe the people around us care much less than they actually do. Loneliness makes us view our existing relationships more negatively, such that we see them as less meaningful and important than we would if we were not lonely.

These distorted perceptions ripple and create self-fulfilling prophecies. If you are feeling emotionally vulnerable, do you convince yourself that people don't like you or aren't interested? Do you hesitate to reach out, fearing being seen as needy or desperate? This might begin to harden you. Perhaps you notice you start to respond to others' bids for connection with you with scepticism, hesitance, cynicism and resentment – effectively pushing away the very people who could ameliorate your loneliness. As a result, you might find that you further withdraw and isolate to avoid disappointment or rejection: 'I won't go to that party, no one will talk to me anyway' or 'I won't ring that friend, they are getting sick of hearing from me' are repeated on a loop. So, what does overcoming loneliness look like?

Loneliness isn't the kind of problem that can be resolved overnight – it takes sustained and conscious effort. Fundamentally, it involves challenging your first thoughts and those gut feelings that keep you isolated and withdrawn. It involves manageable risk-taking. You can make a start with these five things:

1. KEEP A LOG OF WHEN YOU ARE FEELING MOST ALONE

Make a note of the triggers, times in the month, particular dates, times in the day, events in the year, when you feel most alone. Jot down what might trigger your sense of loneliness and, in equal measure, what can ease it and support you to feel better. Are any of the following triggers for your feelings of loneliness?

» Not being invited to a party.
» Sibling dynamics within families.
» Parents separating.
» Feeling overwhelmed at work.
» Feeling tired and unable to part take in social events.

» Other people getting married, having kids, going on holiday.
» Not feeling able to really say how you feel.
» A death or loss.
» A relationship ending.
» A new house, a new job or a new city (or just a big city).
» A birthday (big or small).
» Having a baby/children transitioning away from you/empty nest.
» Not having enough money.
» Not having enough sleep.
» Not having enough contact with people.

There may be smaller, more micro moments of loneliness you can list for yourself. If you can begin to notice your patterns, you can then prepare to support yourself at times you know might be most difficult.

2. DESTABILISE YOUR LONELY FEELINGS

Write down some of the thoughts that you have when you are lonely. For the purpose of this activity, try to amplify them – make them more dramatic than they actually are (ugh, this might be hard to do but it is so worth it):

» 'I will always be alone.'
» 'I'm lonely because people don't like me.'
» 'I'm lonely because I'm not thin/cool/smart/funny enough.'
» 'If I am alone, I can only feel lonely and unhappy.'
» 'I must be a loser, because I am alone.'
» 'No one else feels lonely like me.'

Next, challenge yourself to reframe them in a way that might show you something else about the situation you find yourself in, and lead you into deeper discovery about yourself. For example:

» 'I will always be alone, if that's what I choose.'
» 'I'm lonely because I don't like myself and expect to be alone.'
» 'I'm lonely because I'm unsure what I have to offer others.'
» 'When I am alone I can do things to nurture myself.'
» 'I must be very afraid of people, which is why I'm alone.'
» 'Everybody feels lonely sometimes.'

Next, try to turn them into affirmative actions that will move you away from you feeling stuck in your loneliness:

» 'I am going to choose to be less alone.'
» 'I am going to find ways of liking myself.'
» 'I am going to find ways of showing others my value and theirs.'
» 'When I do these things to nurture myself I feel less alone.'
» 'People have their own challenges and I'll be less judgemental of them and me.'
» 'I'm going to ask others about feeling lonely and share my experiences, even if it's a bit uncomfortable.'

Refer to what you've written as a map for yourself. Try to chart any progress you notice and any meaningful conversation you do have. Notice the times when you feel less lonely and what components were involved. Notice when you come up against your own resistance or challenges ('This is crap', 'It's hopeless', 'This isn't helping') and what led to you feeling that.

3. GO AGAINST YOUR GUT FEELINGS

Commit to overcoming loneliness by going against your gut feeling and challenging those distortions. Challenge that inner voice telling you to play it safe by self-isolating. The fear of rejection can be crippling and paralysing, but on the other side of that fear could be grounded, genuine connections waiting for you to press into them. Statistically, it looks like we're all lonely together, so you reaching out to others might be received as a relieving, comforting, flickering light in the darkness of these times.

4. ACTIVELY SEEK MEANINGFUL CONNECTIONS

Reach out, today, to three people you have had safe connections with before and suggest a catch-up. Does this feel scary, uncomfortable or awkward? This is all understandable, but do it anyway and give them the benefit of the doubt. It is fair to say that if they enjoyed hanging out with you before, they will enjoy hanging out with you now. If they haven't called, don't assume it is about you. As a culture, we often become out of touch with each other – ironically, sometimes even more so in the super-connected world we now live in (busy lives, work and competing priorities all take up our valuable time). Try to recognise that you aren't always the reason for there being a loss of connection.

5. BE OPEN TO (AND MODEL) INTIMACY

One way to encourage deeper connections and more intimacy from others is to express more ourselves. Not everyone will be able to meet us where we are at, but some will, and sometimes we are only able to know that if we model it ourselves and see what we get back. Express positive sentiment and avoid accusations. Focus on the longing, not on criticising the absence. For example, change: 'We just don't spend any time together anymore' to 'I really wish I had more time with you.' Change: 'You haven't called me in months!' to 'I was thinking about you, let's grab a drink or have dinner.' Change: 'You don't even show an interest in what's going on for me' to 'So much has been happening, I'm really looking forward to catching up with you and finding out what's going on for you'.

Connections with others, being able to feel safe with others, is one of the single most important aspects of maintaining good mental health and beating loneliness. Safe connections are fundamental to meaningful and satisfying lives.

THERE IS POWER AND GROWTH TO BE FOUND IN SOLITUDE

The difference between being alone and loneliness is that our aloneness is a choice; we actively pursue moments to be by ourselves. Anything that we feel we have a choice in is useful for our mental health. Choose to be alone sometimes.

Some of us find it hard to be alone, on our own. Do you find the lack of distraction while being on your own frightening? We need to be alone sometimes – to be with ourselves, to rest, to reflect, to find our own balance. Being alone can be a deeply rejuvenating, healing and creative experience. Solitude can be calm, centring and grounding, and it's really important for mental maintenance. If we allow ourselves moments of solitude in the chaos of our daily lives and let the noise around us settle, we can reflect on what's happening in our lives and simply 'be' in a world that is constantly about doing, doing, doing.

Sometimes our own noise can be deafening when we are alone and this can feel overwhelming. Try to stay with it and know that those few minutes that we take to simply be, feel or practise gratitude, can be really grounding and renewing. Here, we can show up more authentically as ourselves.

It's so important to seek meaningful connections in life and focus on those relationships that serve us, but it's also vital that we avoid the traps of comparing ourselves with others and people-pleasing to the point of burnout. Let's discuss that in the next chapter.

Chapter 14

The Comparison Trap

Self-worth is at the core of our very selves – our thoughts, feelings and behaviours are intimately tied into how we view our worth and value as human beings. We constantly measure our worth, but we're often not aware of how we do it; for a lot of us, our self-worth is developed through comparisons. We size ourselves up against others on appearance, how much money we have, how well we please others, who we know/our social circles, what we do/our career, our relationship status and our achievements.

Comparing ourselves to others is a natural human tendency – we're hardwired to evaluate ourselves by looking at others. Sometimes, we compare ourselves to others who we deem as worse off than us. Here, we often come away thinking: 'Well, at least I'm not them. At least I'm here and not where they're at. At least I've got this . . . done that . . .' This usually gives us a little self-esteem boost – in these moments we feel better about ourselves and better about how our lives are going.

Other times, we compare ourselves to others who are seemingly doing better than us. They've got the job, salary, status, partner, kids, house, car or whatever else we want or use as a marker of success. From here, we often come away thinking: 'If I was there, and not where I am now, I'd be . . .', 'If I had that, my life would be . . .' or 'I'll never get there.' This can leave us with feelings of inferiority, dissatisfaction, guilt and jealousy.

Both comparisons have their advantages. Comparing ourselves with someone who we feel is worse off is a quick and easy way to feel better about ourselves. Comparing ourselves to someone who is seemingly in a better position than us can motivate us to want to do better and offer something to aim towards. But both will eventually leave us feeling like shit. The first because relying on other people being in a worse position than us offers quite a shaky foundation for our self-esteem (and there's always a chance of things worsening for us). Comparing ourselves negatively is built on false ground as we typically compare the worst we know of ourselves, to the best we presume about others.

JOURNAL PROMPT

» Who have you compared yourself to in the last 24 hours? Think of the last time you checked your social media feeds. Which posts made you feel envious or as if your life isn't as good in comparison? In turn, did any posts make you feel smug or better than that person?

> » Do you compare yourself more to people you don't know online or people you know personally in real life?
> » Do you compare yourself in a general way, across a number of different areas, or do you have a specific topic that triggers you, like home, work, money or love?

Dealing with Life's 'Milestones'

The intensity of our comparisons spikes around significant time periods: after university and approaching 30 being incredibly common times, especially for women. When you were a kid, we imagine the idea of becoming a 30-something-year-old was a totally abstract concept. Even in our early 20s, when many of us spend a lot of the time recovering from hangovers, scrubbing wine out of carpets/clothes/our soul or moving from job to job, we think that by the time we turn 30, we will have it sorted. But then it approaches. And towards the end of our 20s, abstract ideas about how 30-year-olds should be feel like they're suddenly turning into looming concrete expectations about how we should soon be living our life.

For so many people within our clinical practice, at around 30 years old, buying a home or having a baby are no longer distant things they might want to do one day when they have the time or money – they become achievements that they feel like they needed to have nailed yesterday. They're fuelled with urgency, panic and often paralysing fear that they will be left behind as all their friends march down the cobbled streets to adulthood, while they watch from their Instagram feeds.

As real as the pressure can feel, it is important to remember that you don't need to rush to pull together a life that resembles some other person's idea of how a 30-year-old should live. It is OK to challenge the narratives that are assigned to us at such early ages. For example, culturally, we view property ownership as a maturity ritual. But this maturity-related high wears off quickly – ownership or the accumulation of things doesn't equal happiness. Marriages aren't necessarily a sign of maturity, or a shortcut to stability. Having a baby doesn't make you a mature grown-up, just as not having a baby doesn't make you an irresponsible slacker. Age 30 is not the cut-off to have decided either way, on any of these.

Let's take the pressure off. Most of us are still trying to work it out, even at 40. Turning 30 can bring a lot of positive changes into our lives – we have less time for everyone's bullshit, we tend to prioritise what is important to us, and we definitely spend less time stressing over ambiguously worded text messages.

WHAT LIFE SHOULD LOOK LIKE BY THE TIME YOU'RE 30
However you want it to look! We need to challenge the idea that we need to be a home-owning, child-rearing, dog-walking, married person to be happy, successful and fulfilled (unless you want those things of course).

You Are More than Your Work

In today's world, we expect more than ever from our workplaces: to give us money, freedom, belonging, autonomy, agency, direction, something to believe in, space to be creative . . . We want to feel seen, valued, heard and included. Work has become so much more than making a living; we go there to make friends, make a community, make a lifestyle and make meaning.

Work gives us the means to create the safety upon which our lives depend; it feeds and shelters us and those we love, it gives us a reason to get up in the morning and it can give us purpose. But work can also be the source of so much of our suffering.

There are clear factors that contribute to our suffering at work. It could be that your workload does not match your capacity, leaving you with little time to rest, recover and recharge, which can leave you feeling resentful and exhausted. It could be that your boss is constantly contacting you with an expectation that you'll always be 'on', leaving you feeling out of control with no autonomy. The company's values might not align with yours, leaving you feeling demotivated, which can undermine your mental health. If you're from an under-represented community and your workplace shies away from conversations around race, diversity and inclusion, you'll quickly feel isolated and that you are not able to make yourself heard, which can leave you feeling demoralised. It could be that your pay doesn't match the amount of effort and time you put in, leaving you feeling undervalued and underappreciated. Any of these can lead to chronic stress and burnout, make anxiety and depression worse and knock our mental health off-kilter. (See page 320 for a list of resources where you can access support.)

We could go on, but we imagine you get the point. While these work matters are incredibly difficult to navigate and painful to experience, this stuff is often at the surface – we don't even have to scratch it to see it going on within organisations all around the world. When it comes to our complex relationship to work, there are also often deeper, messier forces at play, both collectively and individually. These forces can be both sources of suffering and catalysts for positive change and growth.

WHAT WE'RE REWARDED FOR

Thinking about work on a collective level, there is a disconnect between what we are rewarded for in our society and in our workplaces, and what is actually good for us. Time and again our workplaces reward those behaviours that can be so incredibly destructive – with money, status, promotions, appreciation and success. Usually these behaviours relate to chronic overworking – we get praised for 'going the extra mile', for our commitment, drive or ambition. 'Skipped lunch? Well done for getting that project across the line!', 'Spent the weekend working? At least you'll be all caught up for the week ahead!'

We have somehow normalised – and even praise – busyness addiction. As a consequence, there is enormous value placed on achievement and productivity. On their own, these aren't bad things – both can serve our mental health in positive ways – but because they are treated as the be-all and end-all, it is unsurprising that you might find yourself being struck with guilt if you feel like you're doing nothing. You might be led to believe that keeping busy is the only way to achieve success. As a result, it's unsurprising that you might feel anxious when you aren't busy, as it feels like a form of failure when you don't have your schedule filled up. This is the kindling that starts the fire that eventually burns out.

TIME FOR REFLECTION

Ask yourself these hard questions:

1. Why are you pushing yourself so hard?
2. What needs are driving you? Is it the need for love, safety, belonging or something else?
3. How is working serving you? What are you avoiding?
4. What anxieties are you holding about what others will think? Do they belong to you? How much of it belongs to the culture that you are a part of?

Work needs to be a part of our lives, not our whole lives. This is because work is, and companies are, incredibly fragile. It makes it a very shaky foundation on which to place all of our self-worth.

A DIFFERENT LOOK AT WORK-LIFE BALANCE

Burnout can have us wanting to put our 'out of office' on and take a forever nap. It doesn't have to be that way. Just by saying 'work–life balance', we put work in *opposition* to life. The fact is that work is a fundamental part of life; who we are and what we do merge – sometimes with good results and sometimes with bad. It can be more helpful to think about it in thirds:

»   One-third for taking care of you.
»   One-third for taking care of your mental and physical health.
»   One-third for your family, friends, work, community and the world at large.

The real gift is learning to be present in whatever third you're living. So, when you're working, work. And when you're loving, love. And when you're eating, eat. Be here now. Below are some ways in which you can find better balance.

Don't be the source of your own stress

We are too hard on ourselves. We 'should' ourselves too often; we strive for perfection and punish ourselves for not achieving it. Give yourself a break. You won't always feel productive or

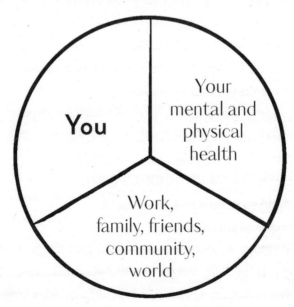

Alternative to work–life balance

creative – the last thing you need to add to your lofty expectations is a layer of shame and guilt.

SIGNS YOU'RE OVERCOMPENSATING AT WORK

» Email psychology: You overuse exclamation marks, people-please and say 'no worries' when people let you down. You go through your emails self-editing your enthusiasm so you fall on the right side of 'likeable'.

» You find yourself saying 'yes' and agreeing to do things much more than you're comfortable with. You are afraid to say 'no' because you don't want to be seen as difficult.

» You're often quiet when you should be raising your voice. You feel nervous relaying your ideas to your team in group settings, either through fear of rejection or you're sick of sharing your ideas only for others to reframe them as their own.

What would you add to this?

Be aware of bad stress

Good stress is a burst of energy that advises us on what to do. It's motivating, short-lived and helps us meet daily challenges. Bad stress is chronic, long-term and leads to an inability to concentrate. Bad stress can mean getting ill more often with colds, body aches and headaches, trouble falling asleep or staying awake, changes in appetite and getting more angry, irritable or anxious than usual.

Notice toxic workplace dynamics

Feeling a lack of control over your work? Do you have unclear job expectations, dysfunctional workplace dynamics, lack of social support? Have you been told you should think yourself lucky that you have a job or feel that way? These are all things that can lead to you feeling exhausted and burnt-out at work. Seek support, voice concerns and/or have a get-out plan.

Know what drives you

Do you feel stuck on a treadmill of overcommitment? Ask yourself: Am I doing all of this because I want to or need to? Or am I doing all of this out of compulsion or fear? Did your parents prioritise and celebrate achievements over emotional connection? Are you overworking to keep busy and distract yourself? Are you over-working as a defence against feelings of not being good enough?

SEVEN TIPS FOR OVERCOMING IMPOSTER SYNDROME

Self-doubt can really hold us back in the workplace. Addressing our 'imposter syndrome' means giving ourselves permission to fully accept that we deserve our success. It means expanding, instead of making ourselves smaller.

1. **Take stock of your successes.** Remind yourself regularly of your successes in order to put together a

strong argument against your feelings of self-doubt. Keep a list of tangible, demonstrable achievements. Ask others for input and go back to it when you feel doubtful of your own ability.

2. **Let go of perfectionism.** Perfection is unrealistic and it will cost you your joy. None of us will ever 'know it all' and none of us can lead mistake-free lives. Set yourself realistic, achievable and challenging goals. Know that progress beats perfection every time. Trying to be perfect all the time can keep you in a cycle of shame, insecurity and low self-esteem.

3. **Aim for 'good enough'.** The phrase 'good enough mother' was coined by Donald Winnicott, a British paediatrician and psychoanalyst. Winnicott observed thousands of babies and their mothers, and he came to realise that babies and children actually benefit when their mothers fail them in manageable ways. Take this concept into your work and aim to be good enough. Make space for mistakes and allow yourself the gift of learning from them.

4. **Resist making comparisons.** Avoid comparing yourself to others. Instead, keep your eyes on your own work. Become who you are. People who spend the least amount of time comparing themselves to others in terms of creativity, career progression or money, also report the least amount of self-doubt, anxiety and regret. When you compare yourself to others, you get hooked on external validation.

5. **Reframe negative self-talk.** Notice when your inner voice is becoming your inner critic. Consider whether your thoughts are empowering or disabling and reframe your scripts. For example, instead of thinking, 'I'm the wrong person for this role', retrain yourself to think, 'I have a lot to offer in the position.' Instead of, 'Someone could definitely do it better', affirm to yourself, 'I am just as capable as anyone else and I worked really hard to get here.'

6. **Know that imposter syndrome has no advantages.** A lot of people dress up imposter syndrome as something positive, something that keeps them humble, hard-working and motivated. But, imposter syndrome is not what drives you or sharpens your craft; instead, it holds you back and stops you from enjoying the things you do. It keeps you anxious and unable to integrate positive experiences after your achievements, keeping you in a negative cycle of self-punishment.

7. **Reach out to others.** Your experience of imposter syndrome is not isolated; you may think it is only happening to you, but you are not alone. Reaching out to people who respect you, who care about how you're doing, will ameliorate feelings of loneliness and disconnection that come with imposter syndrome. You will be surprised how many of your colleagues, mentors, bosses, friends and family (who may also be intelligent, articulate and competent) experience very similar feelings of self-doubt.

Cover the basics

Burnout is a result of too much energy output and not enough energy self-invested. It's pouring from an empty cup and straying too far from ourselves. You know, the mental maintenance stuff we covered in Part 2 that we know helps but that gets thrown out of the window when we're stressed and in survival mode: Have you drunk enough water today? Do you need an early night? Have you had good food? Have you been outside and stretched? Have you been in contact with those you love? Revisit Chapter 5 to ensure you're laying all those important foundations.

SIGNS YOU SHOULD LEAVE YOUR JOB FOR YOUR MENTAL HEALTH

No amount of money, alignment on vision, staff yoga or free lunches can compensate for a dysfunctional, toxic and poisonous workplace culture. Know when to hold on. Know when to let go. Sometimes letting go is the best thing we can do for our mental health.

» You have clearly communicated your needs and nothing has changed.
» You're experiencing chronic stress and no support is in place.
» You constantly dread work.
» It regularly keeps you up at night.
» You are burnt out and this is the company norm.

> » You've stopped caring about your performance.
> » Your relationships outside of work are suffering.
> » You're undervalued and undercompensated.

You are more than your job, your wage or your title. It's okay if you work for a living instead of living to work. Your self-worth isn't determined by what you do.

How to Escape the Comparison Loop

For most of us, the first thing we touch in the morning is our phone. We wake up and, before we've even been to the toilet, we scroll, stopping to pause on a snapshot of the 'perfect' life. We're assaulted 24 hours a day with carefully curated, filtered photos and heavily edited updates of other people's lovely lives, families and promotions. And yet we know those photos are a tiny, manipulated fraction of a life we don't really know anything about.

Though it's our innate human nature to compare ourselves to others, we've never lived in a time in which we could do it as easily as we do, for as long as we do and to as many people as we do. The impact of which ranges from straightforward dissatisfaction and envy, to a wilting self-esteem, anxiety and depression.

Now, unlike the millions of blog posts or six-week coaching courses you can find online, we are not going to tell you to stop comparing yourself to others. This is near-impossible and unrealistic. Comparison is human nature. But what we are going to do is invite you to bring your comparisons closer for investigation. To be curious about them and bring them into the light of day so that they can be challenged. Because of the frequency we find ourselves playing out these comparisons, it is important to remember that the people who you're comparing yourself to, you don't really know very well. What that means is that you see their shiny and curated outside, but you don't see the reality of their life. Don't be fooled by what you see on someone's socials or LinkedIn, and be careful of who you are comparing yourself to.

What we've learnt from our years of clinical practice is that people have hard and complicated lives – even people who seem very fortunate. Often the 'ideal' that we're observing, the one that fills us with jealousy or resentment, is a facade that we create with our fantasies about them. In these moments of comparison, what we're focusing on is their highlight reels. We are not seeing their 'behind the scenes'. This can be found in the story of the CEO who works 90 hours a week, doesn't see their family enough and missed their kids growing up. Or the Managing Director who found all their meaning and value within their work and got to 40 and desperately wanted children and a partner.

When you're stuck in a comparison loop, remember that you are different to other people. They are not like you. They don't have your upbringing, your family, your history, your challenges, your abilities . . . they don't have all of the beauti-fully complex parts that make you up. Only you have those. So, a more healthy and worthwhile comparison is you yesterday versus you today. Focus on that.

Even if you feel your life has taken a step back, say, you're in the midst of redundancy, and you feel that the 'you' yesterday was in a better position than the 'you' today, this approach is still a more helpful comparison than comparing yourself to someone else. Think about what that you yesterday was feeling like, what their situation looked like. Now think of ways in which you might get back there. Is it a new job? What is the first step that you can take towards getting there?

TIME FOR REFLECTION

This is an exercise (creative arts psychotherapy style) we might use within our practice. It offers the chance to take a bird's-eye view of your life. It is an opportunity to be creative (focusing on process, not product) and to be playful. Using found objects, collage, paper and pens, create the following images. Don't get hung up on how your pictures look; feel free to stick, draw, paint and create anything that comes to mind when you ask yourself these questions:

1. **Where you have been:** What have been your struggles? Where have you come from? What are your highs and lows? What moments in your life did you think you might not have been able to get through, but did? What have you survived, overcome and faced?

2. **Where you are now:** Who and what surrounds you? What is in your life right now? Mark people, places and things. What areas have flow? What areas feel stuck?

3. **Where you want to be:** How close or how far away
   is this image from the last? What changes would you
   make to the last? Have a goal and break it down into
   smaller, manageable parts. Aim high, but choose steps
   with a reasonable probability of success. Incremental
   progress, a little better each day, is what you need for
   sustainable growth. Not big leaps, not dramatic life-
   altering changes . . . Small steps like this go a long way.

Once you have done this, create a fourth image of
every resource (internal and external, personal and
social) you have that will support you to get to where
you want to be.

To have good self-worth, we don't need to be perfect. We only
need to accept ourselves as we are at this moment in time and
see ourselves as a whole, despite whatever we may feel we are
lacking. It's about approaching ourselves with compassionate
curiosity. It is about knowing that:

» your to-do list
» your job
» whether you have children or not
» your social media following
» your age
» your appearance
» the amount of money you have
» other people

» how much you go to the gym
» the number of friends you have . . .

. . . are all things that do not determine your self-worth.

Instead of chasing things that temporarily boost our self-esteem, the challenge is in measuring our self-worth by who we are at our core.

Stop Your Inner Critic from Chatting Shit

We have two voices inside of us: one that is nurturing and lifts us up and one that is critical and weighs us down. But for a lot of us, the inner critical voice goes overboard, berating, shaming and finding faults. The inner critic is loud and sometimes overbearing, making the inner nurturer small and ineffective. It wears down our mood, confidence and resilience. We can reset this balance by restraining the critic and strengthening the nurturer inside ourselves.

BE CURIOUS

It can be easy to hate our inner critic, but some of the time it is trying to protect us from feeling like a fraud. It is important to question where it comes from. Does it remind you of anyone – a parent, sibling, relative or teacher? Who is the source? Too often we internalise the words of one person and let that be the narrative that we tell about ourselves, to ourselves and to others. Stepping back from the criticism to observe it can stop reinforcing it and help you dis-identify from it.

'I'm a bad person' or 'I'm a fuck up' – any definite label like this is your inner critic speaking. Notice dismissals or minimisations of your pain, your needs and your rights. Notice the downplaying of accomplishments. It's all your inner critic talking. When we notice it, we can challenge it.

TIME FOR REFLECTION

Let's look at how you can tackle your inner critic and 'kill it with kindness'. Write down one of your inner critic's typical lines (for example, 'You are not good enough'). Now write down three or more believable statements to counter this. For example:

» 'I know you're being harsh and trying to keep me stuck, but I know I am enough. I am enough. I am enough exactly how I am.'

» 'I'm not perfect, but nobody is.'

» 'I am learning, I am becoming and I am unbecoming. This takes time and I am going to be gentle with myself.'

CALL ON YOUR INNER SUPPORTERS

Our inner critic can be made up of a 'shitty committee', so, instead, think about who is in your nurturing committee. When your inner critic gets loud, imagine encouraging people in your life with their hand on your shoulder, imagine them standing behind you. What are they saying? Tune in to this.

WHY WE FOCUS ON THE BAD SHIT
AND HOW TO STOP

As humans, we can't help but focus on the horrible stuff. But we can help ourselves to stop and think, 'Is this helpful?'

We remember bad experiences, insults, criticism and discomfort much more than positive ones – we're hardwired to do so. This is an evolutionary hand-me-down from our ancestors. Back then, alertness to danger, aka 'the bad shit', was a matter of life and death. We needed to remember which tree would be full of juicy fruit and which could poison us.

This irritating phenomenon is called 'negative bias'; when faced with an intensely negative moment and an intensely positive moment, we come away focusing on the negative.

Negative bias will have you going into a job review, being told you're doing an amazing job but coming out of it feeling low, focusing on the one piece of constructive criticism that was given to you. This can lead to devastating dents in our confidence. So, what can you do?

» Question: Is this thought accurate? Is this thought helpful?
» When you notice that negative thoughts or images are starting to enter your mind, imagine a stop sign or try to actually say 'Stop!' to yourself.

» Combat the negative thought by leaning into it. Write it down, rip it up and watch it lose its power.
» Talk to people you trust and ask their opinion. Sometimes we need support to challenge our internal critic.

The more time we spend comparing ourselves to others, the less time we spend on appreciating our own journey, recognising how far we have come, how much we have done to get where we are now. Every second spent looking at everyone else's highlight reel and comparing ourselves to those carefully curated versions of others, we rob ourselves of moments in which we can validate our *own* journey. Despite every challenging moment, every obstacle and every struggle, you are here now. You've endured and survived. You are intrinsically valuable just as you are right now, in this moment and in all future moments on this earth.

At a time of radical self-reliance and independence, we must remember social connections as the most important factor in our mental wellness. Being socially connected is the one thing that saves us from even the most severe mental and emotional challenges – it does so by interrupting that voice that convinces us that we are alone.

Chapter 15

Honouring Your Potential

For us, 'honouring your potential' is about living with an openness to a wide range of emotions, both positive and challenging, and working through them without denial but with acceptance. It isn't about unsustainable self-improvement or constantly overworking – it goes deeper than that. It goes beyond being successful at work, your bank balance or your status. Honouring your potential is essentially living a fulfilled life. It is living with a sense of good-enoughness. It is about finding daily moments to rest, to be present without being tormented by the tyranny of the past or a need to control the future. It is about our internal worlds being as close as possible to our external presentations, to the person that people meet when they see us. It is about feeling aligned to what we feel and trusting these feelings to guide us, and being able to challenge them when we need to. It is less about knowing, but allowing ourselves *not* to know. It is less about learning all of the time, but unlearning. It is about moments of *duende*, the Spanish word, which is one of those untranslatable words but essentially means a spontaneous and creative force, when a fullness of being is experienced, allowing experimentation with the unknown.

What do you think when you hear the word 'potential'? Do you think of striving, reaching or fulfilling? Do you think of following your dreams, thinking big, self-sufficiency, productivity, never settling, relentlessly pushing yourself to the top of your game? This is the language of our time and we don't have to look far to see how we have become so fluent in it. You can't visit a co-working space without being hit by a neon sign imploring you to 'Hustle Harder'. You can't open Instagram without seeing 'Rise & Grind' quotes celebrating a 5am get-up to own the day and 'If you have money and time, you have everything'.

This is hustle culture, drenched in toil glamour, where 'honouring your potential' means ambition, grit and never stopping – often at the cost of meeting your most basic needs. But it's not always as obvious and overt as this. There is a kind of self-help hustle culture that can be found in excessive engagement with online courses, workshops, retreats and seminars. It can be found in devouring #TherapistsOfInstagram quotes and, ironically, collecting piles of books like this one that are then left unfinished or half-read. Excessively and constantly engaging in self-help, driven by a need to perform, to always self-improve and better yourself all of the time, is not only exhausting, but is getting in the way of you actually honouring your potential.

When we're always planning to make the next improvement, we aren't stopping to notice all of the work that has been done. When we're always in action, we leave no space to receive the gifts of insight that come to us in moments of stillness or quiet. When we're always talking, we're not taking time to listen. When we treat ourselves as home renovation projects, and not human beings, we will forever find faults and refuse to embrace the unavoidable reality that we are, indeed, wildly messy human beings and there is beauty in this. So, before we can look at honouring our full potential, we need to look at our limits.

> When we're always looking to what's next,
> there's not much space to be with what's
> already here, right in front of us.

Embrace Your Limits

Take this moment as an invitation to stop and to shift gear. As much as getting outside of our comfort zones and leaning into discomfort can be great agents for change and growth, actually recognising and understanding our limits is one of the most powerful things we can do in honouring our potential. Limits are liberating too. Recognising your limits doesn't involve always reaching or pushing, striving or excelling, but sometimes stopping, pausing, slowing down and remembering who the fuck we are.

We all have individual limits that are rooted in our make-up and are informed by our life experiences, opportunities, knowledge, skills, and so on. Universal human limits include our need for regular and consistent sleep, food, water and sunlight. Less obvious human limits include our need to have fun, play or to be idle. A lot of us have a hard time accepting these limits. We do so because we don't see them as natural, but instead confuse them with weakness. We see limits as flaws, signs that we are not capable and somehow not good enough – and, therefore, we deny the reality of them. But when we constantly deny and fight our limits, feelings of stress, frustration and self-criticism increase. This is because by denying our limits, we often don't notice (until it's too late) when we are being pushed beyond them.

For example, if you know you are a person who needs to fully switch off from work for longer than a week at a time, and you reach the end of the year without booking in a proper holiday, you will no doubt feel exhausted, stressed and resentful. These are understandable, legitimate feelings. Because you have denied your limitations (such as needing more than a week off), you may very well find yourself treating such feelings as illegitimate. You might shame yourself for feeling exhausted, you might feel weak for feeling stressed, you might feel guilty for feeling resentful. Now you are carrying an additional layer of feelings about your feelings. This layer becomes a block from having genuine self-compassion. So what do you do instead? You work until you're burnt out or until you're forced to stop. This then might become an annual experience, a pattern.

So, what is the alternative? An alternative is accepting and embracing the reality of our limits. When we accept them with mindful recognition and self-compassion, we can start to live with more ease and less strain. Less caught up in stress, frustration and self-criticism, we can find ourselves more in a place of groundedness. This looks like recognising that needing a proper holiday is absolutely normal. It looks like recognising those difficult feelings or distress caused by not taking a break as legitimate, worth giving a shit about, worth turning towards (not away from), worth saving yourself from. It looks like stopping. It doesn't sound sexy, it doesn't sound overly ambitious, but it will save you from a lot of struggle and emotional distress.

From this place, we can spend less time on relentless self-improvement and more time on self-acceptance and self-compassion. This is an important part of mental maintenance – the part that recognises that there's a time for doing and a time for being. A time for action and a time for pausing. A time for holding on and a time for letting go. A time for doing the work and a time for resting. A time for churning the soil, for digging deeper and a time for letting things take root and grow.

While there is something to be said in growing through discomfort, we need space to grow. We need to know when to stop, to let the light in. To get some fresh air, to keep ourselves topped up with the things that nourish us and give ourselves space to grow.

Accept Your Messiness

To find your absolute best self you need to give yourself a break from trying to perform, to optimise yourself all the time. Being obsessed with looking inward and trying to achieve your ideals might actually be leaving you less equipped to own and accept your inherently messy, complicated and forever unfinished parts.

This looks like sticking your middle finger up to messages telling you that you're supposed to be happy all of the time. It means knowing that this is a pretty hard thing to do when we're constantly being told we can do and be better, and more positive, and more productive. It looks like arriving at an understanding that self-improvement is a process without an end, a journey with no final destination. Knowing that there will never be a day when you can say to yourself: 'Wow, I've reached my full potential. I am finally the bee's knees, the best, shiniest version of myself.' It is the trajectory, not the position, that is most important. It's where you're heading.

It is a recognition that yes, striving for things is part of being human, but if you only feel OK when your endorphins are coursing, and when you're striving, developing, moving, then you're not really OK. Because from this place, we can never really say to ourselves: 'I am enough. I am valuable. I lead a meaningful life. I don't have to keep pushing myself and striving to be someone else overtime.'

Explore Your Potential

Let us offer you an alternative to the productivity-driven, all-or-nothing approach to goal-setting and self-improvement. We want to offer a gradual path to honouring your potential, on which there are no shortcuts, but incremental, sustainable change. There is hard work, over the long haul, but this is what it takes. Let's start – you will need to grab your notebook:

IDENTIFY YOUR GOAL

This can be an outcome you want, a place you want to arrive at or a change you want to make: 'I want to have a healthy relationship', 'I want to live a more fulfilled life', 'I want to stop engaging in behaviours I know are harmful to me.'

EXPLORE THE MOTIVATION FOR YOUR GOAL

Write a brief paragraph on why you are motivated to achieve this goal. Journal your responses to these questions:

» Why do you want to do this?
» Who else benefits from your achievement of this goal?
» If you were lying on your deathbed and had not attempted this, how would you feel?
» Are you doing this for you or for someone else? (Neither is wrong but you should be aware.)

EXAMINE THE BROADER IMPACT

Write a brief paragraph on how achieving this goal would change your life or help you grow. Consider the following questions:

» How would achieving this change your view of yourself?
» How would it change the way others see you?
» Are there any societal/familial/organisational benefits in achieving this goal? How would it positively impact others?

SET MILESTONES AND DAILY TASKS

This is where you build in feedback and accomplishment.

» Establish a weekly/monthly milestone. Being able to feel like you are making progress and point to milestone achievements is essential to positively moving forward with recognition, care and compassion.
» Break the goal down into action steps. Focus on process instead of outcome. Say you want a promotion at work, a process action step would be to gather all of the data/info you needed to support that conversation with your boss. The next would be to arrange a meeting. These are steps within your control. Schedule time for when you will complete these steps.

IDENTIFY THE MOST LIKELY OBSTACLES AND CREATE SOLUTIONS

Write out 5–10 of the most likely obstacles and develop solutions for them. Draw on both internal resources and external resources. For example, if the problem is you are too tired from work to focus on building healthy relationships at the end of the day, your internal solution might be to factor in more rest. An external support might be to tell a friend you want to see them and would like them to support you in making this happen.

KNOW THAT IT IS THE JOURNEY THAT IS MOST IMPORTANT

Deadlines can be helpful, but our humanness lies not in arrival, but in being almost there. This is what keeps us going, sticking close to the journey, walking towards the selves that we want to be, stopping every now and then to recognise just how close we already are to that self.

Grinning digital yogis, meditating Insta-monks, multitasking mums with no stretchmarks or bags under their eyes – all of these characters who play centre stage on our social media platforms make perfect look achievable. As a result, messy, real-life shit has become dissatisfying, disappointing and undesirable. But by striving for success and perfection all of the time, we miss out – we miss out on our true potential and this bungling, gorgeous, contradictory, heart-breaking paradox we call life.

Conclusion
So How Are You Really?

We've covered some testy stuff in this book and we can't imagine that it has been an entirely easy read. Perhaps it's been grating in places, difficult to imagine yourself in some of our thoughts and ideas as we've reflected on the past. Perhaps you've wanted to slam shut the pages, pour a glass of wine or flick immediately to Netflix (we have too at some points). Perhaps you've come across antagonising, hard-to-read ideas. You might have collided with your grief, your despair, your stuckness. Or perhaps something you've read has given a much-needed voice to some of your feelings, salved some grazes . . . or maybe none of the above!

Whatever your experience, here we still are, together, as we navigate this last chapter, where it feels relevant for us to return to where we began and our belief as humans and therapists – that there really is no easy, quick, neat, one-size-fits-all prescription for continued good mental health. It isn't something that can be simply addressed once, checked off a to-do list, never to be returned to again. A bid for our better mental health is hard, often monotonous, daily work as we try to understand ourselves more fully. It takes commitment to stick with it even when it feels useless. It takes determination to stay with a process that often feels deeply uncomfortable, uncertain and unknown.

At times where it feels like the only thing to do is retreat back to where we've come from (the comfort of the uncomfortable familiar), you'll need to hold on to a speck of belief that you are worth the work, that everything is a process and that you deserve to feel differently, to have more internal space to process and understand yourself a little more. That it is worth staying dedicated to your mental health even when it feels most adverse.

> When it comes to being in good mental
> health, quick fixes are bullshit.

This stuff is not easy – know that plants growing up through concrete did not arrive there without challenge. That there is pain (sometimes months and years) before the courage to change is fully felt, but that when you get there, even in those small increments, it feels good, really good; like coming up for air after a deep dive, or leaving the gym after a session, or the feeling in your body after a stretch. There is a little magic on the other side and it is worth fighting for. You are worth fighting for.

ROAD MAPPING THE FUTURE

Take a pen and some Post-it notes, postcards or magazine cuttings (perhaps even some string, flowers and pebbles, if you can find some), and create yourself an actual map. Have a play with visualising your future:

» Where are you right now (perhaps put yourself in the picture using a photo if you have one to hand)?

» Who and what is in your life with meaning – think of both the positive and the negative? (Use objects, toys, postcards or photographs to symbolise these if you want to.)

» Where would you like to be in 3, 6 or 12 months, or 3, 6 or 12 years (put markers or notes on the image)?

» What is standing in your way (you can use stones and rocks to represent obstacles if you'd like to)?

» What or who is helping and supporting you? Think about internal and external factors. (You could use toys or flowers to represent these.)

» What do you need more of to overcome the obstacles?

Use string or draw lines between the objects and images to show flow and knots. There isn't any right or wrong way to do this activity – just have a play around. You can move and change things, play with taking the things you don't want off, looking at it close up and from far away.

Ask yourself:

» What do I notice?
» What do I like?
» What don't I like about what I see?
» How can it help me move forward?

You can either leave it as an active piece, coming back to it whenever you feel stuck, or take a photo of it.

Practise Self-Compassion

As you move towards an invitation to 'do' more, to work hard and actively participate with yourself, know this . . . **you deserve and should expect love in abundance.** Even when you are struggling, stuck, angry and feeling ugly, you deserve love. The place you can reliably return to over and over for this type of love is yourself. Show up for yourself, meet yourself with some compassion (like those awkward hug/clap yourself moments at the end of exercise classes). Try to create a little bit of space to celebrate your worth and to know you are trying your best. Visualise a younger, less-equipped version of you and feed them a useful nugget that this wiser version of you has discovered. Embrace the younger you with kindness and enquiry and encourage them on.

Stay Curious

The key component to our better mental health is self-knowledge, so enquire fiercely about yourself. Think of yourself as your own user instructions, manual or travel guide – within your pages live all of those self-generated challenges and most of the solutions. You play all the characters and are in charge of the entire narrative (even when you feel you aren't). You might find you need to read and reread sections over and over to make some sense of the words. With self-knowledge and self-questioning – the what, the why, the how, the 'who me?' – comes the possibility of a different, more conscious future.

Grow Through What You Go Through

Some days, good mental health will feel possible and some days totally impossible, and there will be an entire range in between. Because you are multifaceted and made up of moving emotional parts, every day, every hour, every minute you will feel different. You are too complex and extraordinary to be built for continuously feeling good. If you were, you would be without your own incredible depths and would lack the immense propensity you have for empathy towards others. You are built to adapt, to change, to learn and grow from what you go through. We are built to practise, to fail, to keep trying and, from that, keep developing.

Finding ways to feel 'more OK' is personal and unique. We will each develop our own techniques that help us do better and coping strategies for when we don't. Like building muscle, these will develop over time. With the right combination of internal and environmental factors, the more we practise and the more we return to ourselves to enquire, the more successful we'll be.

JOURNAL PROMPT

» Where are you at with yourself now?

» With your parents/carers?

» With your thoughts about feelings?

» About us and what we've suggested and shared?

» How are you really doing?

We All Feel a Bit Shit Sometimes

At Self Space we try as hard as we can to run the company in line with the way we practise therapy. Our values contain authenticity, compassion and hard work, among others. We don't always get it right, but as a benchmark we try as often as we can to connect to our integrity, both personally and collectively. We start every meeting as we start most therapy sessions with the question 'How are you?' We ask once and listen to the answers and then we ask again, 'So how are you really?' Sometimes the answers are the same, sometimes poles apart. Sometimes we hold it together on the first ask, giving neat answers about the weekend, and by the second round sometimes tears are flowing or we say 'we don't know', 'we aren't sure, not so good'. We revert to noises and gestures which depict something yucky or messy, or bleurgh. We have become fairly well-versed now in how little we gain from not answering honestly even if the answers are incomplete, incoherent or hard to say.

We have become so adept at brushing this question off we choose from our library of prepared answers:

» 'Pretty good you know.'
» 'Not bad, busy weekend.'
» 'All good. House is coming on.'
» 'Tired but OK.'
» 'Ready for a holiday but all right.'
» 'Can't complain.'

The list goes on . . . What are your generic answers? All of them act as a way of closing down the question, moving away from an intimate conversation, moving on. They serve no other purpose other than their duty of words. They don't encourage you to be seen and the listener isn't included in your narrative. We all know it's lip service and yet this is what we do, isn't it?

If you sit in the reception of a busy office you'll hear the question thrown around millions of times. Sometimes it's ignored or the user has walked off before their answers have even been spoken. With consideration to what we spoke about in Part 1 (pages 13–96), where we might have come from – sometimes grown, sometimes dragged – let's all consider how we ask and how we answer this question and how we listen to the answers.

What better way to get connected by our messiness? Allow the question to land. Go back to it again and notice what different answers emerge. Explore your unique and connected humanness. Notice how messy, confusing and conflicting the responses are. Do not jump to rescue yourself or them. Do not try to fix, change or even make sense of what is being said. Know that we are all inexplicably messy. We were born messy and we'll die messy. We are smells and fluids, we are bruises and itches, sticky, imperfect parts. We are hopeful and depressed, we are certain and confused, we are awful and beautiful, we are all of it. We are human.

PAVE THE WAY FORWARD

Make some micro promises to yourself right here and now to keep yourself on track:

» Note the things you would like to change. Identify the support you'll need to do it and the steps you'll take to get there.
» Mark and honour your progress, even small steps. Celebrate your progress.
» Stay connected to your value and worth.
» Put Post-it notes in this book to remind you of the parts that resonated and return to them often.

JOURNAL PROMPT

Make a scrapbook of quotes, images and stories that inspire and encourage you onwards. Here are some of our favourite quotes:

» 'Keep going, even though it is taking longer than expected.'

» 'When we strive for perfection, we end up missing out on life.'

» 'Someone's inability to love you is not a reflection of your ability to be loved.'

» 'Saying no to things that make you feel like shit is a heroic act of self-love.'

» 'Choose people who are good for your mental health.'

» 'You will have bad days but they will end.'

This Isn't Goodbye

One of our clients always asks us not to say goodbye at the end of a session – she says it's too final (there is a lot in that!). She asks instead that we say, 'See you.' She tells us that the statement means many things: that we see her, that we'll be seeing her, that we'll hold her in mind, that we'll still be here when she returns. There is a looseness to 'See you' that means that what has happened in the room can follow her outside, it doesn't cease in meaning as the door closes, but it flows with her as she moves on. She takes a little of the essence of our time together with her into her life. We feel that. There is a time and a place for goodbyes, but not right here and now.

With gratitude and love,

See you x

Resources

Birth Trauma Association
A charity that supports women who suffer post-traumatic stress disorder (PTSD) after birth.
01264 860380
www.birthtraumaassociation.org.uk

British Association for Counselling and Psychotherapy (BACP)
The professional association for members of the counselling professions in the UK.
01455 883300
www.bacp.co.uk

CALM
A free and confidential helpline and webchat for anyone who needs to talk about life's problems.
0800 585858
www.thecalmzone.net

Crisis
The national charity for homeless people.
www.crisis.org.uk

Cruse Bereavement Support
The UK's leading bereavement charity.
0808 8081677
www.cruse.org.uk

Mental Health Foundation
The UK's leading charity for mental health.
www.mentalhealth.org.uk

Mind
Provides advice and support to empower anyone experiencing a mental
health problem and campaigns to improve services, raise awareness
and promote understanding.
0300 1233393
www.mind.org.uk

NHS 111
Offers general health information and advice and help for your symptoms if you're not sure what to do.
111
www.111.nhs.uk

Relate
The UK's largest provider of relationship support.
www.relate.org.uk

Samaritans
Offers listening and support to people and communities in times of need.
116 123
www.samaritans.org

Self Space
A contemporary mental health service offering a good conversation with
a qualified person, through straightforward access to flexible therapy.
www.theselfspace.com

Shout Crisis Text Line
If you're experiencing a personal crisis, are unable to cope and need
support, text 'Shout' to 85258.

Notes

CHAPTER 1: WHAT IS 'MENTAL HEALTH'?
MHFA England, 15 Oct. 2020. Mental health statistics. Retrieved from https://mhfaengland.org/mhfa-centre/research-and-evaluation/mental-health-statistics/

CHAPTER 3: ALL THE FEELS
Jung, C. G., 2014. 'Christ, a symbol of the self'. In *Collected Works of C. G. Jung, Volume 9 (Part 2)*. Princeton University Press.

CHAPTER 4: CHILDHOOD MATTERS
Changing Minds, n.d. Donald Winnicott. Retrieved from http://changingminds.org/disciplines/psychoanalysis/theorists/winnicott.htm

Felitti, V. J., Anda, R. F., Nordenberg, D., Williamson, D. F., Spitz, A. M., Edwards, V. and Marks, J. S., 1998. 'Relationship of childhood abuse and household dysfunction to many of the leading causes of death in adults: The Adverse Childhood Experiences (ACE) Study'. *American Journal of Preventive Medicine, 14*(4), pp. 245–58.

Hays-Grudo, J. and Morris, A. S., 2020. *Adverse and Protective Childhood Experiences: A developmental perspective*. American Psychological Association.

Stern, D. N., 2018. *The Interpersonal World of the Infant: A view from psychoanalysis and developmental psychology*. Routledge.

Winnicott, D. W., 1991. *Playing and Reality*. Psychology Press.

CHAPTER 5: THE FOUNDATIONS

Deschasaux-Tanguy, M., Druesne-Pecollo, N., Esseddik, Y., de
    Edelenyi, F. S., Allès, B., Andreeva, V. A., Baudry, J., Charreire,
    H., Deschamps, V., Egnell, M. and Fezeu, L. K., 2021. 'Diet
    and physical activity during the coronavirus disease 2019
    (COVID-19) lockdown (March–May 2020): Results from the
    French NutriNet-Santé cohort study'. *The American Journal of
    Clinical Nutrition*, *113*(4), pp. 924–38.

Jacka, F. N., O'Neil, A., Opie, R., Itsiopoulos, C., Cotton,
    S., Mohebbi, M., Castle, D., Dash, S., Mihalopoulos, C.,
    Chatterton, M. L. and Brazionis, L., 2017. 'A randomised
    controlled trial of dietary improvement for adults with major
    depression (the 'SMILES' trial)'. *BMC Medicine*, *15*(1), pp.
    1–13.

Woodward Thomas, K., 2015. *Conscious Uncoupling: The 5 Steps to
    Living Happily Even After*. Yellow Kite.

CHAPTER 6: PROPER SELF-CARE

Deacon, A., 2004. *Beegu*. Red Fox.
Winnicott, D. W., 1991. *Playing and Reality*. Psychology Press.

CHAPTER 7: ROUTINES AND RITUALS

Ironside, V., 2011. *The Huge Bag of Worries*. Hodder.
Jung, C. G., Von Franz, M. L., Henderson, J. L., Jaffé, A. and
    Jacobi, J., 1964. *Man and His Symbols* (vol. 5183). Dell.
Khodarahimi, S., 2009. 'Dreams in Jungian psychology: The use of
    dreams as an instrument for research, diagnosis and treatment
    of social phobia'. *The Malaysian Journal of Medical Sciences:
    MJMS*, *16*(4), p. 42.

CHAPTER 9: DEALING WITH CHANGE

Jung, C. G., 1970. *Collected Works of C. G. Jung, Volume 11.* Princeton University Press.

Jung, C. G., Von Franz, M. L., Henderson, J. L., Jaffé, A. and Jacobi, J., 1964. *Man and His Symbols* (vol. 5183). Dell.

Samuel, J., n.d. *A living loss: The art of finding and losing yourself* [podcast]. Retrieved from https://juliasamuel.co.uk/podcasts/a-living-loss

CHAPTER 10: DIVORCE AND SEPARATION

McLeod, S. A., 2010. Stress and Life Events. Simply Psychology. Retrieved from www.simplypsychology.org/SRRS.html

CHAPTER 11: WHY WE NEED TO TALK ABOUT GRIEF, DEATH AND LOSS

Jung, C. G., 1983. *Collected Works of C. G. Jung, Volume 13.* Princeton University Press.

Klass, D., Silverman, P. R. and Nickman, S. L., 1996. *Continuing Bonds: New Understandings of Grief.* Routledge.

Kübler-Ross, E. and Kessler, D., 2014. *On Grief and Grieving: Finding the Meaning of Grief Through the Five Stages of Loss.* Scribner.

Stroebe, M. and Schut, M.S.H., 1999. 'The dual process model of coping with bereavement: Rationale and description'. *Death Studies*, 23(3), pp. 197–224.

Tonkin, L., 1996. 'Growing around grief – another way of looking at grief and recovery'. *Bereavement Care*, 15(1), p. 10.

Yalom, I. D., 1980. *Existential Psychotherapy.* Basic Books.

CHAPTER 13: NAVIGATING RELATIONSHIPS

Campaign to End Loneliness, n.d. The facts on loneliness. Retrieved from https://www.campaigntoendloneliness.org/the-facts-on-loneliness/

Colonna, J., 2019. *Reboot: Leadership and the Art of Growing Up*. HarperCollins.

Frankl, V. E., n.d. BrainyQuote.com, BrainyMedia Inc. Retrieved from https://www.brainyquote.com/quotes/viktor_e_frankl_121087

Hanson, R., 2013. *Hardwiring Happiness: The New Brain Science of Contentment, Calm, and Confidence*. Harmony.

Perel, E., n.d. Retrieved from https://www.estherperel.com/

CHAPTER 14: THE COMPARISON TRAP

Winnicott, D. W., 1960. 'The theory of the parent-infant relationship'. *International Journal of PsychoAnalysis*, *41*, pp. 585–95.

Acknowledgements

With thanks to our incredible team at Self Space, the therapists and everyone behind the scenes. Thanks to all of the clients who have shared themselves with us over the years. To Leah Feltham at Vermilion for holding our hands, Julia Kellaway, our brilliant editor, Emma Wells at design studio Nic&Lou, and the team at Penguin Random House.

Jodie: Elivs, Biba and Oscar for your constant support, creativity and tolerance of my absence; Maxine for endless love; Stacey for keeping the light on; Mannie Sher for his expert clinical knowledge and guidance; James Biddulph and Pascal for reading pages of nonsense; the Browns for early belief in everything Self Space; my family for vibrancy and love; and thank you Auntie, for showing me that there is always a choice and that, above all, kindness is the key.

Chance: To Sonny, this is for you boyo. Out of all of the feelings that you'll feel, I hope loved is one that stays with you. With thanks to Mim for the light that shines from you and on to me. It lifts me, even in my darkest days. The space you make for me has definitely helped me grow through the things I've gone through. Thank you to my family, friends and every teacher who believes that 'naughty kids' deserve second and even third chances.

Index

Note: page numbers in **bold** refer to diagrams.